East Meets West
Super Nutrition from Japan

By
Hirotomo Ochi, PH.D.

Edited by
Elias Castillo

Ishi Press Internatio
Mountain View

D1119803

Published by
Ishi Press International
1400 N. Shoreline Blvd, Bldg A7
Mountain View, CA 94043
U.S.A.

First printing February, 1989
Printed in Japan

CREDITS:

Cover Design: Ben Lizardi
South Pasadena

Cover Photograph: Robin Robin
Los Angeles

Interior Photographs: Takashi Kaizuka
Tokyo

Chef: Nagako Koide
Tokyo

Dinnerware: ORANGE HOUSE, Shibuya Branch
Tokyo

Typesetting and Layout: The Graphic Express
Mountain View

TABLE OF CONTENTS

Introduction

For centuries the Japanese have preserved an attitude toward life that has remained virtually unchanged despite the introduction of high-technology into their small island nation. Instead of scrapping all its ancient lifestyles, many were overhauled and reformed to better survive in the fast paced, highly competitive world of an industrialized market.

However, some of those lifestyles remained virtually unchanged. They were the colorful temple ceremonies, the hot baths, ancient music and dancing, traditional architecture and Japanese food. The latter very successfully adopted Western items. The result was an enormous success which has made Japan the world's healthiest nation. The intermixing of Japanese and Western foods has created a highly nutritious diet that is unrivaled in the world. Packed with proteins, vitamins and minerals, its success can be seen in the larger and healthier physiques of post World War II Japanese and in extended vigorous lifespans.

It is a diet that is so low in cholesterol that Japan, among the industrialized nations, has the lowest rate of heart disease caused by that substance.

This book introduces you to that exceptional diet. Some items may be strange sounding to you, among them seaweed, tofu made from soybeans, and the shiitake mushroom, for example. Others will be totally familiar, milk, cheese, eggs, bread and rice.

Through careful and detailed explanations you will learn how to adopt that diet for your benefit. The 12 chapters of this book also demonstrate, through American and Japanese research findings, the dangers of Western eating habits. You will learn that the United States has one of the world's worst rates of heart disease and why. At the same time you will read what foods will help prevent heart attack and cancer and how diet can lengthen your life and make you healthier.

You will learn about superfoods within the Japanese diet that carry so much nutrition that no logical person can ignore them. For example, nutritionists consider soybeans a major source of protein and vitamins, but they are virtually unknown as a food in the United States. Recipes in this book will show you how to prepare foods derived from this exceptional bean.

Seaweed is another product that cannot be found in the Western diet. Yet, like the soybean, it is a major part of the Japanese diet. Seaweed is very high in many essential nutrients without being fattening. For instance, did you know that seaweed has been used successfully in Japan and China as a cure for goiters?

Finally, recipes will carefully explain how to prepare some of the most popular Japanese foods, such as miso soup, tempura and sukiyaki.

The information in this book is not just one researcher's opinion, it is based on critical medical research and health histories of millions of Japanese and Westerners. It truly is a meeting of the best of the East and the best of the West.

■

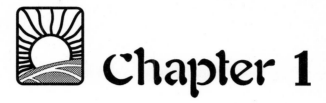 # Chapter 1

The Japanese Way

**Consider the Japanese traditions
of architecture and gardening.**

Both strive for one goal — a harmony with nature in which traditional architecture reaches out toward nature while the Japanese garden sooths by bringing the best of nature into the home.

In the ancient homes, palaces and temples of Japan, the interiors are designed to create an illusion of open space through simplicity. Thus, a large room will not have ornately carved decorations or be filled with stuffed furniture.

Instead, only the barest of essentials — a simple chest of drawers, padded straw mats — will be placed inside. Yet, the effect is soothing as the yellow of the straw mats or a dark, shiny wooden floor blends with polished square wooden beams inside the room.

Large sliding doors, made of translucent rice paper glued to a grillwork of thin wood, allow different shades of light and darkness to permeate the room.

Those same doors may open to reveal a small garden, so simple in its design that it does not challenge the mind but relaxes the viewer in its beauty. It may be composed of only a large, moss covered, rock and carefully patterned sand or gravel with a small twisted tree strategically placed somewhere within the garden's borders.

Again, the effect on the viewer is striking through its simplicity.

These are essential parts of Japanese culture that have grown out of necessity. The islands of Japan are not large, yet they have a population that must live in harmony with its surroundings both manmade and natural. Space is a precious commodity.

There are no immense parcels of land for pasturing cattle and sheep, every acre of rural Japan must be productive either through growing food or as parks, to rejuvenate the mind and body.

So it is with Japanese food.

Long ago, the Japanese realized that if they were to survive in a highly competitive world on an equal basis they would have to squeeze the best out of everything on their island nation.

Through hundreds of years of trial and error, the Japanese diet evolved into one that provided everyone with sufficient calories, not only to remain strong but also to provide enough energy for creativity — the mark of a healthy body and mind.

Take Japan's rebirth after its devastating defeat in World War II. Prior to the war, Japan's industrial might and technology had awed the world. It's engineers rivaled the best in the Western nations and its industrial craftsmen were equal to any in the world.

However, there was a price to pay for this achievement. Life was not easy. Food was in short supply because of war demands. As Japan moved from a mainly agricultural nation to an industrialized country, its diet fell behind. Eating habits which could sustain a rural population were insufficient for the immense stress placed on this population when it was required to produce gargantuan amounts of war materials and industrial goods. Medical care was also not as advanced as in other developed nations.

The average life span of the Japanese was 50 years for men and 53 years for women in 1945. With peace came a revolution in the traditional Japanese diet which adopted the best of Western foods and created eating habits that now produce the world's highest average life span (see chart 1).

Today, through that combination of Western and traditional Japanese food, women in Japan can expect to live 81.4 years and men 75.6 years. Infant mortality has also drastically declined. The introduction of antibiotics also helped increase the life span. Public sanitation was also greatly improved, reducing the spread of diseases such as tuberculosis, which in 1950 was the main cause of death. Today, the probability of a Japanese reaching the age of 65 is 80 percent for men and 90 percent for women.

In today's world an increase in the average life span depends more on older people living longer than on infant mortality. Japan, like America, is becoming an "old-age society" with the average life span expected to surpass today's figures.

The development of these old-age societies began in the advanced countries during the end of the 19th Century. France took the lead and other European countries followed shortly thereafter.

In Sweden, where people live long lives similar to Japan, it took 85 years for the old-age population to increase from 7 percent to 14 percent. Yet, by the year 2,000, Japan's percentage of oldsters will number about 16 percent, all within a span of 55 years.

The Japanese way of life has not only made the country a major economic power, it has also caused a surge to the top rank in the longevity of its people.

How has this happened? Why does Japan's population live much longer and remain healthier than those of other similarly prosperous nations and why does the death rate continue dropping? Moreover, why is the death rate from heart disease and cancer so high in the United States while in Japan it is significantly lower (see chart 2)? The answers can be found in a comparison of Western eating habits with those of Japan.

Eating Customs of the West

In the Western world, food is so abundant that many people overeat, stuffing themselves with sweets, thick steaks, rich sauces and other treats which can harm the body. Such diets are nutritionally unbalanced.

This problem was highlighted by the release of the McGovern Report in 1977. It found that America's health was in danger as Americans feasted on foods rich with fat, sugar and cholesterol. The United States is not alone in facing this problem. All of the advanced Western nations face the same situation.

Three years later, in 1980, another report was issued that sought to modify the unbalanced eating habits of Americans and encourage them, through the following seven suggestions, to maintain good health and longevity.

1. Maintain an ideal weight — obesity is a common factor in adult disease. The best way to maintain an ideal weight is to reduce caloric intake and increase exercise.

2. Decrease the amount of saturated fats and cholesterol — meat and eggs contain a lot of saturated fats and cholesterol and should not be eaten in excess. No more than 30 percent of caloric intake should be in fat.

3. Increase the consumption of starch and fiber. Make up the decrease of fat by eating more complex carbohydrates, such as grains, beans and vegetables.

4. Reduce the amount of sugar in the diet. Sugar is the worst type of food for maintaining an ideal weight. Sugar is the main ingredient in many rich foods and should be severely limited.

5. Eat a variety of foods. To maintain good health, forty different nutrients are necessary. The foods that contain the most nutrients are fruit, vegetables, grains, milk or milk products, meat, fish, eggs, and beans.

6. Cut down on salt. Salt is the main cause of high blood pressure, so it is very important to limit your intake of this seasoning.

7. Don't drink too much alcohol. Alcohol contains a lot of calories but has absolutely no nutrients. Overdrinking is a certain way to destroy your health.

These words of advice are also be applicable to Western Europeans. However, these very important points describe almost exactly the make up of the modern Japanese diet.

For example, while the first point stresses an ideal weight, anyone who followed a Japanese diet would have little problem in maintaining this goal. This is because the Japanese diet is much lower in calories than those of Western nations (see chart 3).

In the Western countries the daily caloric intake is 3,000 calories a day or higher, with the United States and Germany leading the pack with 3,400 calories a day. The Japanese diet, meanwhile, is only 2,600 calories a day.

Fat consumption is also high in the Western world where 40 percent of those calories are in this weight gaining substance. In the United States that figure rises to 45 percent while Denmark is the most unhealthy at 48 percent of calories composed of fat. In Japan, the fat consumption makes up only 27.9 percent of the calories. That percentage is ideal when compared to the 30 percent recommended in Point 2. Japanese fat consumption is low because fish is a major part of the island nation's diet and, in contrast to meat, fish contains little saturated fat.

Another fact that makes the Japanese diet ideal is its percentage of carbohydrate intake which is 59.5 percent. The Western equivalent is 40 percent to 47 percent of total calories. The Japanese figure is higher because in place of fat more rice is eaten in Japan along with soybeans and soybean products. This is in conformity with the third guideline which encourages you to reduce fat and eat more grains, beans and vegetables. In Japan, vegetables are eaten at nearly every meal as recommended by the fourth point. The amount of complex, or unrefined, carbohydrates in the Japanese diet is much higher, and consumption of rich, sugary desserts is much lower than in the West.

Now, while the Japanese diet is low in fat and high in carbohydrates, remarkably the protein level, at 13.1 percent of calories eaten, is the same level as in the West. This is an ideal level, neither too little nor too much. Protein is critical for the body since it is the substance which helps rebuild human tissue in all organs.

Critical to maintaining health is the need to eat many different foods, thus ensuring that we supply our bodies with each of the necessary minerals and vitamins. The Japanese diet supplies this demand of the fifth point. Japanese eat about 30 different foods in their three daily meals and many of these are rich in nutrients.

Finally, Japanese, as suggested in the seventh point, do not consume as much hard liquor as Westerners do. Most adults do not have a cocktail before dinner as is the custom of many Westerners. Instead, beer and Japanese rice wine, called sake, are more frequently imbibed with a meal.

However, while the Japanese diet has many good points it is not perfect. Its most serious shortcoming is that it contains too much salt. This is a problem that can be easily overcome, however, by eliminating pickled foods that the Japanese are so fond of. But still the average daily salt consumption in Japan is only 12.5 grams per person, and this is lower than in the United States. Another point to bear in mind is that only 20% of the population is at risk for developing high-blood pressure because of a high-salt intake. If your blood pressure is within the normal range, you should not overly worry about your salt intake, provided it is not excessive.

When East Met West

Before the end of World War II, the average Japanese was much smaller than persons from the Western world. The reason? An insufficient amount of protein was preventing full development of the Japanese body. This all changed as the Allied occupation of Japan brought with it new foods and a development of a diet that combined the best of both worlds. Kipling may have believed that "East is East and West is West and never the 'twain shall meet." He was wrong.

As Allied soldiers poured into Japan they brought with them milk, butter and cheese, foods that were quickly accepted by the Japanese. And, with the massive burden of a nation on war footing lifted from Japan, the Japanese farmers were able to concentrate on growing more food. The increased production of fresh vegetables, meats, and fish eliminated the great amounts of salt needed to preserve foods. As the Japanese consumed more proteins their physiques also became larger.

With the new diet, Japanese became healthier and lived longer.

One of the first to reap the benefits of this new diet was late Emperor Hirohito, Japan's most revered person who lived into his late 80's. I did some investigation about his eating patterns and discovered some interesting facts.

When the Emperor would arise from the Royal bedroom, he would breakfast on oatmeal, home-made bread, milk, yogurt, vegetable salad and green tea. For lunch he would choose between either a Western style or Japanese meal. For dinner, his chef prepared the opposite of what he had for lunch.

It was a diet that had few calories and his habit of always leaving the table a little hungry contributed to his good health.

Crucial to his eating habits was the large variety of foods he consumed. Among his favorite Japanese foods was rice mixed with barley and fresh raw fish, such as mackeral or sardines. From the West, he developed a liking for dairy foods, meat and meat products and yogurt. All of this food came from his own organic farms and factories where food additives were prohibited.

This is the ideal diet and it is followed by most centenarians in Japan. It is a diet that is low in fat and calories, but rich in nutrients and adopts the best of both Japanese and Western foods.

■

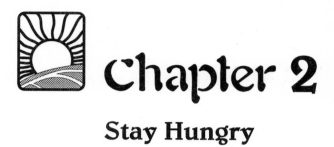
Chapter 2
Stay Hungry

"Ow, I'm so stuffed I couldn't eat another bite."

Those words can easily lead to a lot of pain and suffering if you find yourself repeating them often. Stuff yourself with rich foods and you'll be risking a variety of diseases that will not only make your life miserable but also shorten it.

Sure, you can pig out once in a while, but don't do it often. It's better to follow the Japanese proverb which says that "Leaving the table hungry is the basis of good health." It's an ancient saying, but there is scientific proof that the Japanese knew what they were talking about.

That old standby, the lab rat, helped prove that habitual over-eaters are risking their health. In the 1930s Prof. Clive M. McKay of Cornell University took a bunch of rats, all genetically identical, to see what happens when you stuff yourself.

Here's what he did. After the rats were weaned, one group was fed a normal, well-balanced diet, containing all the necessary nutrients: protein, fats, carbohydrates, vitamins and minerals. The second group was fed the same diet, except that the number of calories in their diet was reduced to near-starvation.

The result was surprising. Instead of becoming sickly, the starved rats turned out to be healthier than those fed a normal diet. In the first group, nearly all the rats had the normal life span of more than three years with the oldest living for 969 days. In the second group, the hungry ones amazingly surpassed their well-fed cousins. Many of the thin rats even lived to be more than 1,000 days old. One oldster reached the ripe old age of 1,465 days — equivalent to a 150 year human life span.

And, don't think that the thin rats were hobbling around on little canes and wheelchairs. It was just the opposite. Prof. McKay found that their bodies were physically young, even at their advanced age. When the normally fed rats were dying like well, rats, the underfed ones were sporting glossy coats, were extremely vigorous and acting like a bunch of sex starved Yuppies. At the age of 1,000 days — equivalent to over 120 years for a human being — they were just entering maturity.

Alright, you may say, that was 50 years ago and science has advanced and maybe today's scientists might come up with different results. Well, guess again. The experiment has been repeated throughout the world since then and the researchers have come up with exactly the same findings. It is, up to now, the only proven way to significantly extend life span in mammals.

Will It Work For You

This does not mean you should start starving yourself. It is critical to emphasize that caloric restriction alone will not cause an increase in life span or keep your hair nice and glossy. In fact, if caloric restriction does not go hand in hand with adequate nutritional requirements, your life span will actually be shortened. That's why people in underdeveloped nations live such short lives.

Originally scientists thought that restricting calories would only work if you started on such a diet at a very early age. Recent experiments have shown that caloric restriction can be effective if begun in adulthood, but the way in which this diet is introduced to the animal is critical.

Scientists have found that the life spans of adult animals can become longer only if calories are gradually decreased over a period of time. If it is done suddenly, the action shocks the animal and life becomes shorter than if the animal had just eaten normally. The trick, to extend life for animals, is to introduce caloric restriction gradually over a period of time, while making sure that the diet is rich in the essential nutrients. And, the earlier in adult life this regimen is begun, the longer the animal will live.

While there is no scientific proof that this type of diet is good for humans, there are many scientists who believe that calorie restricted diets will extend life span. These beliefs are also backed up by statistics. For example, many long-lived Japanese in mainland Japan and Okinawa, particularly, have existed most of their lives on low-calorie, nutrient-dense diets, similar to the underfed rats.

Eating Less and Living Longer in Okinawa

The oldest Japanese are those who live in Okinawa — a chain of islands in the southernmost part of Japan. On those islands are found an incredible number of people who are over 100 years old. While Japan has the world's highest number of centenarians at 2.2 per 100,000, Okinawa has an amazing 10.1 persons 100 years or older per 100,000. In fact, the world's oldest person was 120-year-old Okinawan Shigechiyo Izumi, who died on that island in 1986.

These are not just claimed ages either, they are backed up by carefully kept government records, begun in 1872, that are nearly 100 percent reliable.

In Okinawa the average caloric intake is very low, about 2,100 calories daily for each resident. However, while the caloric intake is low, the amount of animal protein is 203 percent and the amount of green-yellow vegetables eaten is 309 percent more than the national average of all Japan. In contrast, sugars comprise only 26.5 percent of the Japan average.

Even more dramatic is a comparison between the two main causes of death in the United States, Japan and Okinawa (chart 5). For example, major cardio-vascular diseases in America killed 409 persons out of every 100,000 in 1986. In Japan that figure was only 224.8 per 100,000 while in Okinawa it plummets to only 130.8 deaths per 100,000. Figures for ischemic heart disease are even more dramatic with 224.5 deaths per 100,000 in the United States, 40.1 in Japan and a rock bottom 27.8 in Okinawa. Incredible figures indeed.

Blueprinting Your Long Life Diet

Hopefully, you are now ready to accept that a low-calorie diet is the best means of staying healthy. The hard part is trying to find the right foods — rich in nutrients but low in calories — that will enable you to maintain a daily diet of only1,500 to 1,800 calories. Unfortunately, there are few Western foods that meet those requirements.

However, the Japanese have such foods and you can now buy them in many supermarkets. These foods, brimming with essential vitamins and minerals, are low in calories. By combining these low-calorie, nutrient-dense "super foods" with high-quality Western foods you can stretch your life span and enjoy many more healthy and vigorous years. These super foods and their amazing qualities are explained later in this book.

Sumo Wrestler's, Pigging Out and Dying

You've undoubtedly seen pictures of Sumo wrestlers — they're those beefy, gargantuan blocks of fat and muscle who wear a skimpy looking outfit that looks like a baggy jockstrap and grunt and puff trying to hurl their similarly built and attired opponents out of a small ring.

The Japanese go ga-ga over these oversized lard buckets. And well they should, because the life of a Sumo wrestler isn't long. Therein lies the moral of low-caloric intake.

To be competitive, a Sumo wrestler must weigh at least 275 pounds. It's not uncommon to see 350 pound behemoths crunching their way into Sumo rings. In 1988, Japan's top Sumo wrestler weighed an incredible 500 lbs.

That weight is not all muscle either. In order to maintain that enormously unhealthy weight, the wrestlers must gorge themselves with food.

The effect? Some years ago a top-ranking wrestler had to have his appendix removed. He was rushed for an operation into one of Tokyo's best hospitals where surgeons successfully removed the diseased organ. Doctors believed he would have no problem recovering. Yet, within two days the wrestler died. Puzzled doctors could find no explanation for the unexpected death until an autopsy was performed. What the pathologist discovered stunned the doctors — the wrestler's organs were like those of an old man, even though he was only 31 years old.

Sumo wrestlers also rarely live to be more than 50 years old and diabetes is a very common disease among them.

These facts should convince you even more, when linked to those from Okinawa, on the importance of low caloric intake to achieve a long and healthy life.

■

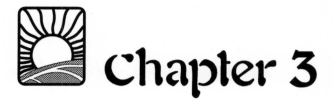

Chapter 3

The Japanese Meal

The Japanese meal is built around rice, the staple food that fills much the same role as potatoes in the United States. Rice is what provides the energy requirements or calories.

The remainder of the dishes, in the typical meal, may contain super foods that are packed with protein, vitamins and minerals plus they are low in calories, reducing the amount you have to eat to get the necessary nutrients.

Like a well balanced American meal, the Japanese meal consists of the staple rice, a main entree, one or two side dishes and soup, usually miso soup. Each dish provides something necessary for your body. Rice, of course, supplies the starch or energy requirements. The main entree provides protein and fats, while the side dishes consist of vegetables providing the necessary vitamins, minerals and fiber. Soup, usually made from miso, a soy bean product, rounds out the meal.

Thirty is the Magic Number

An important characteristic of the Japanese diet is that usually 30 different foods are eaten in the three daily meals. This ensures a well balanced diet plus it keeps the meals from being dull. Of course when we say 30 different foods we don't mean

30 types of dishes but the number of ingredients contained in all the dishes eaten in one day.

Take salads, for example. They usually contain lettuce, onions, tomatos, carrots, bell pepper, and oil and vinegar for the dressing. That is a total of seven ingredients. Eating identical tossed green salads at two meals however will not help provide you with 14 ingredients, only 7. Instead another dish should be chosen to reach the 30 different ingredients.

Thirty ingredients a day may sound like a lot of food, but it really isn't since you'll be eating a small amount of each item. By eating all these foods it's a guarantee that you will be getting all the necessary nutrients each day. In later chapters I will give you specific menus and recipes, plus nutritional information for a number of Japanese dishes and planning Japanese style meals.

Why a Staple Food?

As we have said, rice is the staple food for Japan and is the main provider of starch. The Japanese also eat other sources of starch such as noodles, which are called udon and soba. Additionally, sweet potatoes are eaten in Okinawa.

The Japanese eat some bread as well. Of course, in the Western World, bread is served at nearly all meals. However, bread's role in the Western diet cannot be compared to that of rice in Japan. In Western meals, bread simply compelements a meal. In some meals, bread may not even be served as a side dish.

It's a different story in Japan. Rice is served at all three meals. It is usually served plain with no seasoning and is an important factor that keeps Japanese from overeating. For one thing, it expands and fills the stomach, giving a sense of fulness.

Rice also keeps you from overeating rich foods. You can easily eat a 14 ounce steak when you are hungry. But with rice, you can cut that amount in half and still be satisfied. The rice, instead of the steak, will have filled your stomach. Moreover, if you eat a bite of rice, a bite of meat, then a bite of vegetables, you won't concentrate on just one food. This way you can satisfy your appetite before you overindulge in a single food.

Rice also has another advantage over bread. Rice takes longer to digest so that the feeling of fullness and satisfaction will last much longer after each meal. Rice also comes in small kernals that must be chewed more carefully. Bread, on the other hand, is made from wheat flour which is milled into a fine powder which, after it is baked, is quickly digested. You can eat a lot of bread, but the feeling of fullness will not last long.

Having a staple food is necessary because it prevents you from overeating. Without a staple food, everything becomes a staple and you wind up stuffing yourself. People who like to eat meat usually eat it until they are completely filled with meat. But meat is not a very filling food so you tend to eat more of it, as well as more calories and fat, than if you had eaten a staple food.

That's how people get fat. Their appetites are good so they wind up eating their favorite foods. People who like steaks tend to have them in many meals. These are the people who ignore other foods or eat them in such small amounts that all their meals are nutritionally unbalanced. Instead, they eat a lot of fat and calories they never burn up. They're the ones who become overweight and suffer heart disease or other illnesses associated with obesity.

Why Rice is Good for You

You've learned that rice can satisfy you and keep you from eating too much of a rich dish. But did you know that rice also has protein. While rice contains a lot of starch, 100 grams of boiled rice contains 2.6 grams of protein.

Here's the protein lineup for different types of rice. Brown rice scores 66 (white rice, 62) where eggs, as the standard, score 100. Compare the rice figures to wheat flour which has a score of 36 (whole grain wheat, 50). It's obvious that rice is more nutritious than flour. Furthermore, rice protein has all the eight essential amino acids necessary to make the other 12 your body needs. The presence of these eight in a food indicates the quality of its protein. On this point, rice is a better protein source than flour. Of the eight essential amino acids, brown rice is short of only lysine, containing only 66 percent of the amount necessary to perfectly complement the other seven amino acids, whereas whole wheat is short of lysine by 50 percent. Keep in mind, however, that the main purpose of eating rice is not for protein, but for starch which your body changes into energy.

Now, you've probably been wondering, can I get fat by eating too much rice?

No. A normal serving of rice, 4 ounces, carries160 calories. An equal amount of bread (about a slice and a half) has approximately 260 calories. Even if you eat rice with each of your daily three meals, you'll only be consuming about 480 calories. That leaves a lot of calories remaining that can be obtained from other foods, even if you are on a diet that allows you only 1,500 calories per day.

And, rice is readily available in the United States. In fact, so much high quality rice is grown in the United States that growers want to export some of it to Japan. California rice is also better tasting than Japanese rice and is even more nutritious because of higher calcium and vitamin B2. Start using California rice as the centerpiece of your meals and you'll have an even better diet than is eaten in Japan.

However, cooking rice can be a problem. It is easy to overcook or undercook rice, make it too watery or too dry. You just cannot boil rice and make it taste good. The Japanese have come up with the right answer after centuries of perfecting the preparation of rice. The secret is the electric rice maker, easily available at electric appliance shops. You'll find one of these in every Japanese home. With the rice cooker you'll enjoy rice at its best.

The Main Entree

In Japan, the most common food served as the main entree is fish. It is eaten several days per week and is one of the healthiest sources of protein and fat.

Many Americans eat too much fat which they get from beef and dairy products. The fatty acids in animal fats are mainly saturated fatty acids and these are precisely the fats that increase the amount of dangerous cholesterol in the blood, causing arteriosclerosis and coronary heart disease.

To counter this, American nutritionists have warned against such eating habits, urging a reduction in animal fats and replacing them with the unsaturated fatty acids found in vegetable oils, which can reduce the amount of cholesterol in the blood. Even that may not be good enough, since over-indulging in foods rich in fats, whether saturated or unsaturated, can lead to heart disease and autoimmune diseases.

Yet, fat is needed by the human body. Fats are part of the membranes of cells, plus they are building blocks, along with protein, in the human body. However, only 1 to 3 percent of our calories need to be in fats, specifically linoleic acid, an essential fatty acid. Without this critical fat we would soon die. So, what is there to do? Eat too much fat and you get obese. Eat too little and you'll become unhealthy.

Fish are the answer. Our gilled friends are rich in another group of fatty acids known as Omega-3. One of the more important of these is eicosapentaenoic acid, usually known simply as EPA. Although an animal fat, EPA can prevent heart disease.

The story of the discovery of EPA is fascinating and begins when a Danish researcher named Dr. Jorn Dyerberg traveled to Greenland to study the relationship between disease and the eating habits of Eskimos. Dr. Dyerberg wanted, in part, to find out how Eskimos, who do not eat vegetables, maintained their health . Eskimos' diet consists mainly of meat and fat from seals, caribou and sardines.

One of the first things Dr. Dyerberg discovered was that Eskimos hardly had any cases of heart disease, even though they ate only meat and fish. He examined 1,350 Eskimos and of those, only three died of cardiovascular heart disease. If an equivalent number of Danes had been examined, 40 would have died from that disease.

The Danish scientist continued his research, studying Eskimos in Greenland, Danes in Denmark and Eskimos in Denmark. The discoveries were amazing.

■ Eskimos in Greenland had high levels of EPA in their blood, but little arachidonic acid (In the body lenoleic acid is changed to arachidonic acid, and high levels of this fatty acid are related to various kinds of heart disease and autoimmune diseases such as asthma, arthritis and diabetes).

■ Danes had high levels of arachidonic acid in their blood, but low levels of EPA.

■ Eskimos living in Denmark showed the same blood profiles as Danes.

Dr. Dyerberg had discovered that Eskimos were brimming with the health giving EPA in their blood because they were getting it from seals, caribou and sardines which make up the main part of their diet. Those very same animals also have high levels of EPA.

His findings determined that eating dark oily fish meat like sardines and mackeral on a daily basis throughout your life will help prevent arteriosclerosis. In Japan, sardines and mackeral are eaten almost daily.

Americans, because they do not eat much of these fish, have almost no EPA in their blood, but the Japanese, who eat fish daily, have significant amounts which cuts down heart disease. Japanese who live in rural farming areas have 28.8mg/100ml of EPA in their blood and have the highest rate of heart disease in Japan, whereas the fishing communities have the lowest rate with 34.8mg/100ml of EPA. The lowest rate of heart disease is found in Okinawa where the consumption of fish is twice that of mainland Japan and Okinawans have 46.8mg/100ml of EPA in their blood.

It is my recommendation, based on this data, that Americans should include fish, especially dark oily fish, in their meals as much as once a day.

Vitamins, Minerals and Fiber

Now that we have discussed the main entree, let's turn to the side dishes. These should consist of dark green vegetables, seaweed, beans and mushrooms which are rich in vitamins, minerals and fiber. Not only are they tasty they add variety to a meal plus guarantee a nutritionally, well-balanced diet.

In Japan, the side dishes are made mainly of vegetables which have been boiled in water and are called ohitashi. Making ohitashi, such as spinach, broccoli, etc., is simple. These vegetables should be boiled lightly then removed and rinsed in cold water. After the excess water is squeezed or shaken out, they are cut and served. Some vitamin C is lost in boiling but the other vitamins and minerals remain. In Japan, ohitashi is eaten with a little soy sauce. Boiling and softening your vegetables allows you to eat five times the amount you could eat than if you ate the vegetables raw. This is an important point since persons living in the Western nations do not get enough fiber, the main reason why cancer of the colon is so common in those countries but rare in Japan (see Chart 6).

And, you can eat a lot of vegetables since they are low in calories. Vegetables are also saturated with water and fill your stomach making you less inclined to overeat. Another plus is that the fiber in vegetables works to promote the excretion of toxic substances from the colon.

Most Western style meals do not provide enough vegetables, but by adding ohitashi in large amounts, you can correct this defect.

Miso Soup

A major part of a Japanese meal is miso soup, served in small, usually black or red lacquered bowls, and made from a paste of soybeans. Next to rice, it is the second most common food served in Japan.

In fact, it is so common that in Japanese prisons, convicts are served a standard fare of rice, misoshiru and pickles. Surprisingly, most convicts come out of prison healthier than when they went in. Naturally, that diet can't take all the credit. Most outlaws overindulge in anything and everything. In prison, the regimented life prohibits that type of life which may be a factor in their becoming healthy. In any case, it shows that miso soup and rice isn't harmful.

Rice and miso soup is a perfect combination. Eaten together they ensure that your body gets all the amino acids needed to build protein your body needs. While rice is a bit short of an amino acid called lycine, miso soup has enough of this substance. And, while miso soup lacks methionine, rice has enough of this amino acid. Therefore, the protein score of rice and miso soup reaches 100 when eaten together at the same meal. In vitamins, white rice is a bit low in vitamin B1, but miso soup carries large amounts of it.

Indirectly, miso soup also adds to the number of vitamins and minerals needed by your body. That's because of the various ingredients used in this soup. For example, you can always be certain of getting all the minerals you need by adding to the soup a seaweed known as wakame.If you feel you need more protein you can add another soy bean product called, tofu.

Remember the super foods I mentioned earlier? Well, tofu, wakame and miso are three of these foods.

■

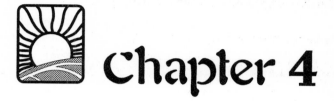

Chapter 4

The World's Top Super Foods

In all the world there is only one vegetable that can be rated as the top super food. That vegetable is the soybean.

Packed into each kernal are all eight of the essential amino acids in high enough quantities to rate a protein score of 100. That's equal to eggs, milk, fish, and beef. No wonder the Germans called it "meat of the fields" when it was introduced to them by the Japanese in the late 19th century. Germany tried to cultivate it, but failed because European soil does not contain a nitrogen fixing bacteria known as rhizobium which is needed to grow the vegetable.

There are three major ways in which soybeans are used. The first uses the whole bean itself, the second uses the high-quality protein of soybeans and the third uses the oils for cooking and salad oils. It is the first two groups that are most used in Japanese cooking.

Japanese have been eating this remarkable vegetable since ancient time because of the influence of Buddhism, which prohibited the eating of meat. The combination of soybeans and rice provided Japan with every nutrient they could have obtained by eating meat.

Not only do soybeans contain proteins, they are also brimming with vitamins B1, B2, A, D, E, along with other special elements. More important, you don't have to worry about fat if you eat soybeans. The oils in soybeans are the unsaturated fatty acids, in contrast to the saturated fatty acids of meat which contribute to high levels of cholesterol. In fact, the unsaturated fatty acids in soybean oil will actually decrease the levels of cholesterol. Moreover, seven percent of the oils in soybeans are in the omega-3 group of fatty acids, the same group in which EPA is found. It is one of the few land-based vegetable sources of the omega-3 fatty acids.

Another nutrient found in soybeans is lecithin. Lecithin has many beneficial effect on the body such as the following:

■ It promotes the normal secretion of hormones
■ It promotes the efficient function of the blood and blood vessels
■ It eliminates bad cholesterol
■ It promotes the absorption of vitamins
■ It promotes metabolism and makes the skin beautiful
■ It controls the increase in peroxidized fats.

Ironically, the United States is the leading producer of soybeans and provides 60 percent of the world's supply, but most of this is used to extrude oil while the crushed leftovers are wasted in feeding livestock.

Soybeans In Cooking

In the summer, Japanese enjoy munching on green soybeans and drinking beer. They're about as popular in Japan as eating peanuts and beer is in the United States. These soybean snacks are a highly nutritious snack that is high in vitamins B1, B2 and C, plus they have appreciable amounts of calcium and iron. In Japan these greenbeans are called edamame and they're made by boiling the beans in water until tender (about 15 to 20 minutes) together with the pods, then rinsed with cold water and shelled. The pod is thrown away (see Chart 7).

Dried soybeans are another rich source of vitamins B1 and B2 as well as calcium and iron. Along with sunflower seeds and almonds, soybeans provide the highest amount of vitamin E (21 mg per 100 grams of beans) that you can get from any other food besides vegetable oils. They also provide fiber. Dried soybeans can be cooked with a number of other foods to make a variety of dishes that are described in Chapter 11.

Still another food that uses the whole soybean is fermented soybeans. These are called natto in Japanese and are usually eaten for breakfast. They do have a drawback, however. Their odor is not pleasing and even some Japanese will turn their noses up at them. Eating natto has to become an acquired taste. Besides lacking a pleasant smell, natto are very high in salt, which means it should not be eaten more than once a day.

MISO. Now we get to miso, the soybean paste from which miso soup is made. Like natto, it is also a fermented food but without the smell. Miso also has an excellent taste. Not only can miso be used in soup, it is also used as a seasoning and can be eaten by itself.

An unusual peculiarity of miso is that research at Hiroshima National University have determined that miso is somehow effective in protecting animals from radiation.

The first inkling of this unique property came after the atomic bomb was dropped on Hiroshima and Nagasaki in World War II. Doctors who attended victims, who were covered with radioactive fallout, suffered almost no ill effects from the radiation emitted by them. Since the only food those doctors ate during that period was miso soup with seaweed, it was hypothesized that one of these two foods may have provided protection from radiation. Recent research at Hiroshima University have provided scientific results that this was a correct conclusion.

In the experiment, four-week-old rats were divided into two groups. One group was fed a standard feed, while the other group was fed dried miso. After one week all the rats were injected with two radioactive elements, iodine-131 and cesium-134. When animals are exposed to iodine-131 it is absorbed by the thyroid gland. Cesium-134 accumulates in the muscles and intestines.

Within 36 hours of being injected, the amounts of these elements in their bodies were measured. Neither group showed differences in the amounts of these elements absorbed in the thyroid glands. The big difference involved the miso fed group. It came when iodine-131 was measured in the blood and cesium-134 was measured in the muscles of that group. Researchers surprisingly discovered that the amounts of both substances were much lower in the miso group.

How and why this works has not been determined but research is underway to discover how miso removes radio-active substances from lab animals.

In Japan, the main seasonings are not salt and pepper but soy sauce, a dark, soybean derived, liquid which has a unique flavor that can enhance the flavor of almost any dish.

SOY SAUCE (and miso as well) does have a drawback. It is very salty but since it is used as a seasoning very little salt is actually eaten. Even if you consumed as much as 10 grams of soy sauce this would amount to only 600 mg of salt. That's far below the recommended daily consumption of 8,000 mg allowed for a healthy person and leaves enough room for other salty foods like miso.

TOFU, the protein of soybeans, is a bean curd made by boiling the beans, crushing them, then collecting the juice and adding a coagulant which turns it into a curd.

Tofu is virtually tasteless allowing it to be mixed with any kind of food, including miso. In miso, soy sauce is added to provide flavor. Japanese enjoy eating it cooled during the summer. In winter, it is boiled and eaten with seasonings and soy sauce. Another plus for this food is that is contains virtually no salt.

There are many varieties of tofu and nearly all of them are available in the United States. Some of them are:

■ Freeze-dried tofu — this is a convenience food that can be stored for a long time. Its nutritional value is the same or a bit higher than regular tofu. When you eat it, boil it with seasoning.

■ Deep-fried tofu — Tofu fried in vegetable oil.

■ Grilled tofu — Tofu pressed with a weight for about 50 minutes then grilled. The pressing gives it a firm structure. This kind of tofu is used in making sukiyaki.

■ Yuba tofu — Made from the membranes of soybean "milk" and then dried.

■ Powdered tofu — This is powdered soybeans. It is used for spreading over rice and for making Japanese cakes. By using a coagulant with it you can make your own tofu.

The nutritional values of tofu are shown in charts 7 and 8 which shows they are rich in vitamins and minerals.

GAMMODOKI, sometimes called Tofu Burgers, deserves special mention. This is a deep-fried tofu made by mashing pressed tofu and mixing it together with sesame seeds, vegetables, and seaweed. It is then kneaded, shaped into balls, and deep-fried. In contrast to ordinary tofu which has a bland taste, gammodoki are quite delicious, with a meaty taste. But this alone would not rate it a listing as a super food. Gammodoki are also high in calcium, iron, and protein. One hundred grams of gammodoki contains 270 mg of calcium. That's in the same category as milk, but without milk's high saturated-fat content.

OKARA is the residue of the crushed soybeans used to make tofu. Unlike in the United States, the Japanese do not dump it nor is it fed to livestock. Okara retains all the fiber lost in making tofu and contains a high amount of protein, calcium and vitamins B1 and B2 (see Charts 7 and 8). Since it contains fiber you can eat it and soon feel satiated without having to eat a large number of calories. Okara is often found in the diet of elderly Japanese.

Seaweed: A Second Super Food

SEAWEED, has always been eaten in Japan. Its export has a fascinating history when during the Edo era (1603–1868) Japan tried to isolate itself from the rest of the world. In those 265 years, the Japanese rulers strictly forbade any contacts or trade with the outside world. However, seaweed became part of goods that were smuggled from Japan into China during those years. The Chinese particularly valued seaweed in treating goiters. It was 100 percent effective because of its high iodine content. All seaweeds have a high iodine content but one particular seaweed, called Kombu, was particularly popular among the Chinese and Okinawans. Kombu was produced mainly in Hokkaido, the northern-most island of Japan, from which the smuggling route was soon established.

While Kombu is eaten by all Japanese, it is especially favored by Okinawans who use it daily and for New Year celebrations plus rituals for birth and marriage.

The most common varieties of seaweed eaten in Japan, besides kombu, are wakame, hijiki and nori which are also sold in most oriental food stores in the United States. Nori, (dried laver), rich in iron and vitamin B1, is the most popular seaweed in Japan. Americans can recognize it as the dark green, thin, wrapping for sushi.

Seaweed has almost no calories yet is one of the best sources of the human body's essential minerals, especially calcium, iron, magnesium and zinc. Additionally seaweed is high in vitamins, has a high protein score, and provides fiber. (see Charts 9 and 10).

Not only must seaweed be considered a super food, it also has been found to inhibit cancer in research with lab rats. The research was launched as part of studies involving the fact that modern epidemiological studies show that cancer rates are very low among people who consume foods high in magnesium. Konbu and other seaweeds are particularly high in magnesium and this may account for low cancer rates in Okinawa where it is eaten in large quantities.

Research findings studying a link between magnesium and low cancer rates were presented at the 1988 International Magnesium Symposium held in Kyoto. There, Prof. Hideki Mori of Gifu Medical School described his experiments with rats.

Mori described how 62 genetically identical rats were injected with a cancer causing substance. The rats were then divided into equal groups. One group was fed hydrated magnesium with their meals, and the other was not. Other than that, the amount of feed they were given was exactly the same.

After eight months the rats were examined. Only 20 percent of the group which was fed magnesium developed cancer while just over half, or 56 percent, of the group that did not receive magnesium developed cancer in the large and small intestines.

Seaweed is also high in other minerals that epidemiological studies indicate help prevent cancer. Selenium is one of them. In the northeastern and northwestern coastal United States, where soils are deficient in selenium, the rates of both cancer and heart disease are higher in those areas than the national averages.

Fish and Shellfish

Now we come to fish. Our scaly friends must be considered a super food like the soybean and seaweed. Why? Because they are rich in a number of vitamins, minerals and are an excellent source of protein with minimal amounts of fat.

In fact, fish should be considered so important in your diet that it should be eaten once a day. As mentioned in Chapter 3, fish is almost the sole dietary source of EPA and omega-3 fatty acids which protect against heart disease.

The darker the meat, the more EPA in the fish. The richest sources of EPA can be found in Mexican anchovies, Atlantic menhaden, mackerel, sardines, herring, salmon, and tuna (especially the fatty parts of tuna). The rule of thumb is that dark oily fish such as sardines, herring, mackerel and salmon are the best sources of EPA.

However, not all fish are high in EPA. Fish which derive their food from sources outside the ocean food chain are usually low in the omega-3 fatty acids. Among these are catfish which contain very low amounts of those acids.

There's even more benefit to eating ocean fish. It is rich in vitamin D, which helps your body absorb calcium, and if you do not drink milk fortified with this vitamin or get sun exposure on a regular basis eating fish is an excellent way to obtain this vital vitamin which is commonly not found in most foods. Another way to obtain this vitamin is by eating certain varieties of mushrooms.

Fish also has more protein than meat while tuna, skipjack, horse mackeral, and salmon are higher in vitamin B1 than beef.

From the ocean, your diet should not leave out shellfish, which include lobster, crab, oysters and clams. These foods provide one of the most concentrated sources for minerals needed by your body. Oysters are an unrivaled source for zinc, containing up to 40 mg per 100 grams of oysters or almost 300 percent of the recommended daily allowance.

Eating shellfish two or three times a week can almost guarantee that you will never suffer from iron deficiency. For example, short necked clams are a concentrated source of iron at 7 mg per 100 grams.

All shellfish also contain appreciable amounts of calcium, comparable to that found in milk. Certain varieties contain 10 percent more calcium in weight than milk.

Shellfish are high in minerals because they absorb their food from the ocean floor and thus do not lack a single mineral. Research has shown that various trace minerals like selenium, manganese, iron and zinc help prolong life. It is probable that the high amount of shell fish eaten by Japanese is another reason for the long lives of these island people.

Shiitake: The Super Mushroom

For 2,000 years traditional Oriental medicine has hailed the mushroom as an important part of its medicine chest. In Japan, the oldest books on traditional healing have references to mushrooms.

These tasty morsels, which can be eaten either raw or lightly stir fried, have a number of outstanding attributes. In Japan, the shiitake mushroom is perhaps the most widely eaten in that nation. It is this mushroom that has been the object of intense research because of its anti-cancer properties.

Experiments carried out on rats at the National Research Center in Tokyo (Cancer Research, Nov. 1970) demonstrated that shiitake contains substances capable of causing complete cancer remission in mice. Researchers discovered that the mushroom contains a substance called lentinan, a highly effective substance in fighting cancer. When 10 doses of lentinan was given to these mice in doses of 1 mg per kilogram of body weight, the cancer was inhibited in 95.1 percent of the mice while 60 percent showed complete tumor remission. At increased doses, such as 5 mg per kilogram of body weight, 70 percent of the mice showed complete tumor remission and the inhibition rate was 97.5 percent.

While lentinan can repress cancer, the exact way it works has not been determined. It does not effect cancer cells in culture so it is believed to work in combination with the body's immune system. Research does indicate that lentinan stimulates the production of interferon, a substance which protects the body from viruses.

Lentinan also has no toxic side effects as do other anti-cancer drugs, nor does it leave scars at the site of tumor remission. Even at extremely high doses of 25 mg per kilogram of body weight, no toxicity was detected.

However, at doses of 25 mg it was less effective in inhibiting cancer, indicating an optimal dose. At that amount, of the 73 percent of mice in which their cancer was inhibited, only 22.2 percent had complete tumor remission.

Also a part of shiitake is a substance called eritadenine which can reduce cholesterol levels and relieve hypertension — one reason why Japanese include this mushroom with high-cholesterol meat dishes.

Shiitake is a good source of all the B vitamins plus ergosterol, a form of vitamin D. Mushrooms are one of the few land-based foods that contain this vitamin. Japanese often eat small fish, bones and all to get calcium. Adding mushrooms ensures a source of vitamin D.

It may be likely that all mushrooms contain anti-cancer substances. For example, mushroom farmers in Japan have lower mortality rates from cancer when compared to the rest of the country.

Little wonder then, that the shiitake mushroom is considered a superfood and should be included in at least one of your daily meals. Shiitake mushrooms are usually available at supermarkets throughout the United States.

Daikon (Japanese Radish): Nature's Digestive Aid

Another superfood that comes from the ground is a radish called daikon which helps digestion through the enzymes it contains. Faulty digestion can mean that your body is not absorbing all the nutrients from the food you eat. Elderly people sometimes find it hard to digest certain foods because their bodies do not secrete many digestive enzymes.

One common example, is the inability of many people to digest milk. However, this can be overcome simply by drinking milk that has been enriched with an enzyme that digests the lactose in milk.

Not only does daikon contain digestive enzymes it also has substances that inhibit the formation in the stomach of nitrosamines, which can cause cancer. The radish is also rich in vitamin A, calcium and iron. By weight it is a better source of calcium than milk. Daikon additionally contains appreciable amounts of vitamins, B1, B2, C and niacin.

The best way to eat daikon is to prepare it raw because high temperatures over 120 degrees fahrenheit will destroy the digestive enzymes. In Japan it is popularly eaten as a grated garnish served with tempura and other oily dishes. Remember, though, to eat grated daikon soon after it has been prepared — the enzymes have a half-life of about 20 minutes.

■

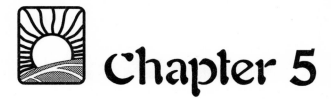

Chapter 5

Western Foods in the Japanese Diet

We have now reached that point where we can discuss those Western foods that have become part of the Japanese diet. The most common of these are milk and milk products, meat, poultry, eggs and bread.

Beginning in the 1950s, the introduction of these products increased the Japanese physique and virtually eliminated any deficiency diseases such as rickets. Yet, because the Japanese traditional diet has not been scrapped, but rather incorporated the Western foods, Japan continued to eat a much lower intake of fat and calories than in the West.

In fact, as more and more Japanese travel and live abroad, markets are now stocking Japanese foods to meet their demands for native foods. Their craving for Japan's special foods tends to keep expatriate Japanese from never straying too far from the eating patterns they learned as children.

As I've said before, I believe that the combining of Western foods with the Japanese diet is the major reason why Japan's senior citizens, are the oldest in the world.

Recently, a dietary survey of people aged 100 years or older was conducted by the Tokyo Metropolitan Government's

Institute of Gerontology. The survey discovered that a variety of Western foods were included in their diets, with 30 percent drinking a glass of milk daily. Additionally, more than half ate high-protein foods such as fish, beef, pork, eggs, soybeans and soybean products twice daily and also ate a hefty amount of vegetables.

Let's analyze some of the Western foods that the Japanese eat. You may be surprised at some of their qualities.

Pork

Pork, despite its popularity, has always gotten a bad rap in the West. Yet, it has been a popular Japanese food for centuries and is eaten with little concern, especially in Okinawa where it is a major protein source.

Just like the Germans, the Okinawans eat every part of the pig, including the feet. However, the difference is that they trim away as much fat as possible and their way of cooking ensures that very little fat is eaten.

Nutritionally, and this may surprise you, pork is superior to beef and is one of the best sources of the B group of vitamins. For example, a serving of lean pork will give you almost 100 percent of the required daily amount of vitamin B1, 29 percent of the RDA of vitamin B2 and nearly 50 percent of the RDA of niacin. Pork liver is also an excellent source of iron for persons suffering from anemia. There is no better concentrated source of easily absorbable iron than is found in pork liver. It contains over three times (13 mg of iron per 100 gram serving) more iron than beef liver.

A serving of pork liver will provide more absorbable iron than from any other food source plus provide the RDA of niacin, vitamins A, and B2 plus many other nutrients.

The trick to eating pork and staying healthy is to simply remove as much fat as possible.

Eggs

Another food that has been given an unnecessarily bad reputation are eggs. That reputation has been given eggs because of their high cholesterol content. Yet, my opinion is that this view is exaggerated because eggs contain three substances — lecithin, choline and inositol — which keep cholesterol under control.

Eggs are also one of the most nutritionally balanced foods available, containing almost every nutrient — the lone exception being vitamin C. And, eggs never seemed to harm Shigechiyo Izumi who lived to be 120 years old. He ate eggs from the chickens he kept several times a week.

The only drawback to eating eggs is that they should not be eaten raw. Uncooked eggs contain a substance known as avidin, which destroys biotin, an essential nutrient. But don't worry about this, you would have to eat more than seven raw eggs daily over a long period of time before you noticed any adverse effects.

Japanese, like Westerners, use eggs in a variety of ways, in soups, custards, omelettes, as well as by themselves. We'll review these dishes later in the book.

Japanese Dishes That Use Western Ingredients

If you've ever eaten Japanese food, you might have ordered sukiyaki in the United States, a mixture of tofu, vegetables and thinly sliced beef cooked in a broth.

This is not a traditional Japanese dish. Instead it is relatively young, having first been concocted 120 years ago when Japan opened up its gates to the West.

Westerners brought beef with them, but not enough to eat thick portions of meat. Steaks were hard to come by, but the Japanese decided they liked beef and so came up with the idea of cooking it in a pot. They named the dish sukiyaki.

The main ingredients for sukiyaki are:

- Thin sliced beef
- Deep-fried tofu
- Vegetables, mainly onions and chrysanthemum leaves which have a strong flavor.
- Shirataki, a starch made from an herb called devil's tongue.
- Shiitake or other kinds of mushrooms
- Soy sauce, in which all the above ingredients are boiled

Other ingredients also used, include Chinese cabbage and burdock. Every item is included to balance nutrition and taste.

For example, since meat is an acidic food, all the other ingredients are alkalinic. Protein is provided by an animal source (beef) and a vegetable source (tofu).

Shirataki, is a zero-calorie food but because of its bulkiness and filling qualities tends to keep you from overeating beef. Even though shirataki is 96.5 per cent water is contains a lot of calcium and even some iron.

Obviously, it's hard to keep from eating good beef, but by cooking small portions with other ingredients, it's taste is picked up by all of them, satisfying diehard beefeaters. Additionally, the soy sauce enhances the flavor even more. A further bonus to nutrition and taste is to dip each bite into the raw egg that accompanies this dish.

In a Japanese meal, sukiyaki is both the main entry and the side dish with rice served seperately as the accompanying starch. One serving of sukiyaki equals 500 calories. If you include the rice and egg, a sukiyaki dinner comes to about 700 calories.

Eating sukiyaki as a main meal has everything going for it. The dish is not high in calories and is well balanced, providing lots of vitamins, minerals and fibers plus protein. Worldwide, sukiyaki is recognized as a healthy, stamina giving dish.

Tempura

Tempura, is another dish with a Western background although its exact origin is not clear. It is believed to have been introduced to Japan by Portuguese traders, since the word tempura seems to be derived from the word tempero, which means "deep-fried" in Portuguese.

It's main ingredients are seafood and vegetables coated with flour and deep-fried in vegetable oil. The heat from frying eliminates the water from the seafood or vegetable, enhancing its taste.

Seafood tempura usually consists of small white fish, shrimp and cuttlefish providing high quality protein without animal fat. The vegetables used are eggplants, sweet potatos, carrots, bell peppers and onion. Fat is provided by the oil used in frying and starch comes from the flour coating. The combination provides you with protein, fats, and carbohydrates, all in one meal. Like sukiyaki, tempura combines the main meal and side dishes in one food. Rice and miso soup can complete the meal.

Tempura should be eaten immediately after it is fried. Eating tempura that has been allowed to stand in the open air allows oxygen to react with the oil, creating toxic substances that damage body cells and your body's DNA. The oil must also be fresh and should never be used more than once.

Japanese radish is the common garnish for tempura and since daikon contains large amounts of digestive enzymes it helps in digesting the oil used in preparing tempura. Grated ginger can be also added and helps in digestion. Both these root plants are mixed in a thin table sauce called tentsuyu, in which the tempura is dipped just before eating.

A standard serving of tempura with soup and rice is about 800 calories.

Tendon is a popular variation of tempura which is very popular as a lunch item among Japanese office workers. It consists of a deep bowl of rice topped with tempura, usually shrimp and is a high-calorie dish containing about 800 calories.

Katsudon, is another popular variation of tempura but with a deep fried pork chop topping the rice instead of seafood.

Other Non-Japanese Dishes

Japanese cooks prepare a large number of foods that are not native to the country but frequently served in homes. Here is a brief list of some of them:

■ Stir fried vegetables — Adapted from China in which vegetables such as bean sprouts, cabbage, leek, chives, carrots, onions and green vegetables are stirred and fried in a small amount of oil until cooked. This is a good way of ensuring that all vitamins in the vegetables are preserved.

■ Meat roasted over open flames-mainly pork and beef and eaten with gravy seasoned with salt and pepper. Adapted from the Korean style of cooking. (I cannot recommend this way of cooking meat, even though widely practiced in Japan, because it produces toxic substances when the flames come in contact with the meat. This will be discussed in Chapter Ten.

■ Eggs — prepared in a variety of ways: fried in butter or vegetable oil, as omeletes or boiled.

■ Potato salad — adapted from the West.

■ Stews — meat and vegetables cooked together. A typical Western concoction.

■ Bread — toasted or used for sandwiches along with vegetables and processed meats.

■ Dairy products — milk, yogurt and cheese.

The next chapter discusses how to combine these Western foods with Japanese dishes to achieve a nutritionally balanced diet.

■

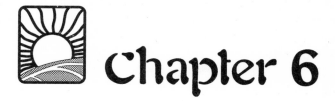

Chapter 6

Balance Your Diet, It's Simple

The secret to a long and healthy life is eating the right foods in the right quantities. While that may be obvious, how do you keep track of the nutrients and calories you need to maintain that goal? Short of becoming a nutritionist, it looms as a monumental task.

There is an easy answer. The trick is to daily eat a large variety of foods selected from four different food groups. You don't eat equally from each of these groups; you eat more foods from some than from others. This method ensures that you will be getting all the necessary nutrients and by including some of the Japanese superfoods also means keeping calories down but maintaining a high intake of vitamins and minerals.

These are the four basic groups and their foods:

- Group One – milk, yogurt and cheese
- Group Two – meat, fish, eggs and beans
- Group Three – seaweed, mushrooms, vegetables and fruit
- Group Four – grains, cereals, nuts and vegetable oils
- Group Five – alcoholic beverages, soft drinks, coffee, tea and sweets.

I wrote about four groups and I've displayed five. This fifth group can be classified "recreational foods" since all they contribute are calories and few vitamins or minerals. There is no need to exclude these foods if you are healthy and not trying to lose weight. However, they should be consumed in moderation and should not become substitutes for any of the foods in the four groups.

Remember, eat these fun foods only after you have satisfied your basic nutritional requirements and with the precaution that they do not exceed your minimum calorie needs.

The reason these foods have been set in four groups is to ensure that daily you eat foods from each of them (excluding the fifth group). Most diets fail because the amount of calories is too low, the diet is nutritionally unbalanced or both. These pitfalls can be avoided by selecting foods from the four groups at each meal.

Food also fulfills a psychological need and the items in the fifth group are those that help make eating a pleasurable experience. Eating can help you achieve satisfaction, but if you cut back drastically and constantly worry about eating, you create tension. This tension develops when, for example, you break a diet and then feel guilty. All people who have lived extremely long lives are happy and relaxed and are never overly concerned about their food.

Izumi, the long lived Okinawan had no qualms about drinking a glass of shochu (a spirit made from brown sugar) every day. Your mental health, which should be relaxed, is just as important as your physical health.

What the Four Groups Do

GROUP ONE: MILK PRODUCTS AND EGGS

Mother's milk is the ideal food, containing every nutrient needed for human health and growth. Unfortunately, breast milk is reserved for infants. Adults have to do with cow's milk, which can be considered a super food since it nourishes calves until they are ready to graze on their own.

Obviously, the main reason to include milk or milk products in your diet is because of the calcium it contains. As much as one third of the women in the United States do not get enough calcium. Many women did not get enough calcium when they were young, a situation that can lead to osteoporosis, the loss of calcium from bone, in later years.

While milk is rich in calcium, remember that it is also high in protein and contains vitamins A, B2, B6, B12, plus every other vitamin and mineral your body needs. Milk sold commercially also has been fortified with vitamin D. The drawback to milk is its high fat content (one glass equals 250 calories). It's best to drink non-fat or low-fat milk.

If you're one of those people who cannot digest milk, substitute yogurt or cheese which are just as high in calcium as milk. However, those products have few of the B vitamins. By eating certain kinds of cheeses, such as Swiss or Parmesan, you can get more calcium per calorie with the same amount of fat as milk. The exception is cottage cheese which, while low in fat, is also low in calcium. The best milk products are low-fat milk and yogurt which have almost the same number of calories as the high-fat products, but are significantly higher in calcium and a bit higher in other vitamins and minerals.

Another reason you might want to include yogurt or cheese in your diet is because it contains useful bacteria which are found in the human intestines.

It may surprise you, but inside your stomach and intestines are more than 400 types of bacteria, some of which are beneficial while others are harmful. The harmful bacteria are normally controlled by the beneficial bacteria, creating a stable symbiotic environment.

An imbalance may occur during an illness in which the harmful bacteria over reproduce. When this occurs, these bacteria release toxins that can cause a variety of diseases that range from simple diarrhea to cancer of the colon.

Yogurt helps maintain the healthy balance in your intestines because the thick, sour tasting, product carries many beneficial bacteria. Two of the most important are bifidobacteria and streptococcus lactis (SL), a traditional yogurt and cheese starter.

Research at the Institute for the Control of Aging in Shizuoka, Japan, has shown that the latter bacteria carries some remarkable properties.

Somehow, streptococcus lactis helps slow down the aging process. In one experiment, two groups of lab rats were fed the same diet of commercial pelletized feed. One of the groups was also fed 120 mg of SL daily. At 27 months there were striking differences between the groups of rats.

The group which did not receive SL showed all the signs of advanced age. Some had curved spines, their hair had thinned and their vascular systems had aged rapidly.

The group fed SL had none of these signs. In fact, they appeared to be as young as the other group was at six months old.

A few of the rats in both groups were also subjected to high doses of X-ray irradiation. Again, the S L group showed less damage than the control group.

Most lactic bacteria live in the large intestines where they control harmful bacteria, but SL is absorbed in the small intestines. This ability to be absorbed in the small intestine apparently is linked to ability to enhance immunity.

Cheese and yogurt carry SL, but this bacteria, which originates in plants, can also be found in corn, lettuce and wheat.

GROUP TWO: ANIMAL AND VEGETABLE PROTEIN

Each meal should contain one serving of an item from this group. For example, you can eat meat at one meal, fish at another and either soybeans or a soybean product like tofu or miso at another.

My recommendation for eating fish daily is because it contains omega-3 polyunsaturated fatty acids like EPA.

By eating about 100 grams of fish, 50 grams of meat and a serving of tofu or miso soup daily, you will be getting an adequate amount of protein while keeping saturated fats to a minimum.

Do not try and get all your protein from vegetables because they do not carry vitamin B12. Obtaining the necessary protein using only vegetable protein would require careful planning that only a professional nutritionist could accomplish. Moreover, certain foods have to be eaten at the same time to allow the different amino acid profiles to complement each other. And as far as being a vegetarian, note that of all the centenarians studied by the Tokyo Institute of Gerontology, there was not a single vegetarian among them.

Besides protein, this food group is a major source of important minerals such as iron, zinc and copper and also contribute a number of other vitamins and minerals to your diet.

GROUP THREE: VITAMINS, MINERALS AND FIBER

Group three, and that includes seaweed, is the major source of your body's need for vitamin C, vitamin A, magnesium and fiber. Foods in the other groups have very little vitamin C or none at all and the daily recommended allowance is 60 mg (by following the meals outlined in Chapter 11, you will be getting more than that each day).

Vitamin A is either obtained from dark green or yellow vegetables or liver (either beef or pork). If these foods are ignored you will not obtain the minimum required amount of vitamin A.

Vegetables also contain magnesium which, as stated earlier, is an important mineral that also protects against cancer. Without adequate amounts of magnesium, calcium cannot be used efficiently by the human body.

Notice that I have included seaweed in this group. Seaweed is not normally eaten in the Western nations, but there is no reason why it should not be included. It is one of the super foods and it is also a vegetable, containing many vitamins and every mineral in extremely high quantities. Additionally it carries a high protein score. Seaweed is now widely available in the United States and should be included in your meals just as it is in Japan and Okinawa.

Fiber is the final reason why items from this group need to be part of your daily eating habits. For many years fiber was be believed to have no significance in healthy living. Then it was discovered that it kept foods moving through the intestines, preventing the buildup of toxic wastes and also is important in the prevention of diseases such as cancer of the colon, obesity and arteriosclerosis.

Consider these beneficial points of fiber if you plan to diet to lose weight:

- It has no calories
- It prevents the excess absorption of sugars and fats
- It prevents constipation
- Controls the amount of insulin, glucose and neutral fats released into the blood.

These foods should be eaten liberally at all meals. At least one of these servings should consist of a dark green vegetable plus fruit. Try to include seaweed in at least one of the dishes that you eat each day. In Japan, bits of it are included in miso and other soups. Seaweed salads can also provide an alternative to ordinary salads (recipes for these are in Chapter 10).

GROUP FOUR: ENERGY AND VITAMIN E

While the first three groups will take care of protein, minerals and vitamins, they will only provide you with a total of 800 calories per day. Another source of energy is needed and that's where rice comes in.

Eating brown rice and whole grain breads will allow you to get the most vitamins and minerals from these group of foods and also provide you with daily calories. They will also supply you with the maximum amount of vitamins B and E.

Japanese rarely eat brown rice, preferring the taste and texture of white rice. However, polished rice is very low in B vitamins, and those who depend on it as their only source of vitamins are in danger of developing a vitamin deficiency.

A healthy trend in Japan is to add barley to white rice. This mixture is called mugimeshi, a highly nutritious food that was popular in ancient Japan. Nearly half of all school lunches in Japan serve rice and barley which is also making a comeback in homes and restaurants.

Mugemishi is excellent for someone on a diet, it has lot of fiber and is low in calories. Another plus for barley is that it carries vitamin E, which makes up for the loss of this vitamin in rice during the polishing process.

Eating brown rice with each daily meal will provide you with less than 500 calories. That amount, plus the 800 calories obtained from the other food groups, will give you a total of 1,300 calories. After this, you can eat almost whatever you like up to the limit of calories you allow yourself daily. Even if you limit yourself to only 1,800 calories daily, you still have 500 calories to enjoy yourself or to make up the few vitamins or minerals that your diet may not be providing you. Just be careful not to overindulge in sweets, alcohol or high-fat foods.

The significance of dividing foods into these four groups is that by eating the appropriate amount from each of them, you do not have to worry about getting sufficient protein, fats, carbohydrates, vitamins and minerals.

Let's consider, the appropriate amount that you should eat daily from these four groups.

CHOOSING FROM THE FIRST THREE FOOD GROUPS

The trick of balancing your diet is to include items from the first four food groups spread over all your daily meals, ensuring that you obtain all the essential protein, fat, vitamins and minerals needed for good health.

From Group one, limit yourself to about 250 calories. Either a glass of low-fat milk or a bowl of low-fat yogurt will total 160 calories. Make up the remainder from eggs, cheese or butter. The milk or yogurt is important since, besides calories, it will provide more than 350 mg of calcium, or nearly half of the RDA. If you don't like milk or yogurt, then substitute them with cheese.

From Group Two, eat a dish of lean beef, pork or chicken at one meal, fish at another meal and then include beans or soybean products in your other daily dishes. The total number of daily calories from this group should not exceed 350 calories.

Include a large amount of vegetables from Group Three in all your meals because they are low in calories. Fruits, however, are usually high-calorie foods (about 80 calories per fruit), so include only one in your core diet. You can eat more as snacks, just as long as you don't exceed your calorie limit.

ENERGY AND VITAMINS FROM GROUP FOUR

Group Four will provide you with your needed daily calories which should not exceed 160 per meal —the amount in a bowl of rice or two slices of bread. Therefore, by eating a bowl of rice with two of your three meals and two slices of bread with the other meal, you will complete the core of your daily diet.

An essential item in your diet are vegetable oils to ensure you are getting sufficient vitamin E plus the minimum requirement of lenoletic acid, an essential fatty acid important for good health. Vegetable oils become part of your diet when you use them to cook foods or as part of salad dressings. Whole grains such as brown rice and whole wheat bread are also rich in vitamin E, but including vegetable oils ensures a healthy amount of this vitamin.

By eating as I've suggested from these four groups, your daily caloric intake should be about 1,500. At this point, eat whatever else you want to complete the caloric intake you have chosen. Rest assured that by using the four groups as the core of your diet, you will eat the right amount of nutrients to stay healthy.

Snacks

Don't forget about snacks. They should be part of your daily diet and can ease those mid-afternoon cravings for food. You can also use them to make up for an item of a food group missed during one of your regular meals. Or, if you are lacking some specific nutrient, eat a food that contains a high amount of it.

Water

You should drink about seven to 10 glasses of water daily and more on hot days. Water helps you stay healthy by aiding in digestion, and helping the kidneys excrete toxic wastes.

Your body consists of 60 per cent water and this amount must
be maintained. Even if you did not eat, but were able to have
water you could live for a rather long time. However, if you
lose 10 percent of the water you will endanger your life. A
20 percent loss means death.

Japanese drink large quantities of water daily by drinking green
tea with every meal and throughout the day.

An Example of a One-Day Menu Based on the Four Food Groups

BREAKFAST

Two slices of whole wheat bread and butter (210 calories)

One bowl of yogurt with strawberries (180 calories)

Vegetable salad —tomato, lettuce, bell peppers, cucumbers
(50 calories)
Total calories – 440

LUNCH

Egg and leek soup (43 calories)

Pork liver with boiled carrots and broccoli (225 calories)

Spinach with bonito flakes (30 calories)

Brown rice (160 calories)
Total calories – 458

DINNER

Miso soup with wakame (30 calories)

Fish iwashi (210 calories)

Stir-fried vegetables (80 calories)

Brown Rice (160 calories)
Total calories=480

Grand total=1,378 calories

Try to determine how many calories you should eat daily. You can do this best by considering your level of activity and energy needs, body size, sex, age, whether you are pregnant or lactating, general health or if you are overweight and dieting to reduce.

Ideally, your daily energy intake should equal the amount of energy used in your daily activities. Avoid an unhealthful situation in which you expend 2,500 calories daily but are taking in only 1,800 daily. When you have insufficient calories available for your energy requirements the body's metabolism rate slows down to compensate. Over a long period it will have an adverse effect on your health. Remember, that there is a limit to how much the body can withstand low caloric intake.

Body size and sex are also important factors in determining how many calories you need. The larger your body the more energy you need to maintain it. Generally, women have lower metabolism rates than men so they do not need as much food as men. That changes when women become pregnant or are lactating, because energy and nutrient requirements greatly increase. During those periods women should increase their intake of high-energy foods and nutrient-rich foods.

Children and teenagers also need tremendous amounts of food, since their bodies are growing and they need enormous amounts of nutrients. Their ravenous appetites should not be curtailed. During adulthood, energy requirements gradually decline.

If you are overweight, try dieting at the 1,500-calorie level until you reach your weight-loss goal. As long as your diet is balanced with adequate protein intake, your excess body fat will be burned up as it makes up for any moderate caloric deficit. Once you have reached your ideal body weight, gradually increase the number of calories until it reaches your energy consumption. This topic is covered in my book **"Dieting Can Ruin Your Health."**

Keep in mind that the quantity of food you eat is related to the length of your life as has been proven in animal experiments. If we are to live past one hundred years in good health, we need to study those who have achieved long life and try to imitate their examples.

■

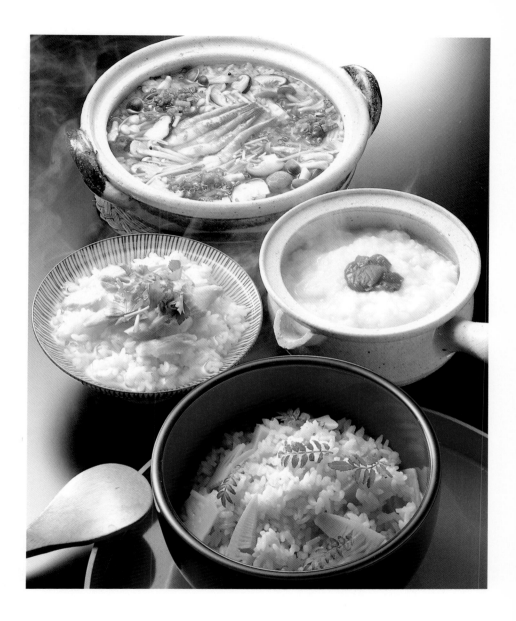

RICE DISHES: Rice and crab/vegetable porridge – OKAYU ■
Salmon ochazuke (left) ■ Rice gruel and umeboshi (right) ■
Rice and bamboo shoots TAKENOKO-GOHAN

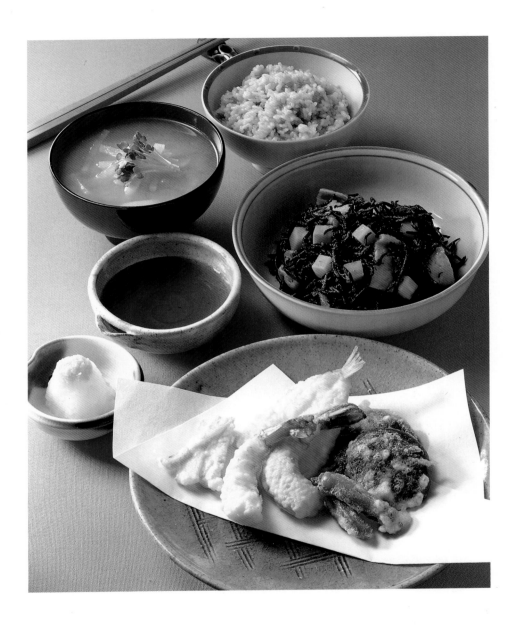

DAY ONE LUNCH: Rice ■ Miso soup ■ Hijiki and sesame
seeds ■ Tempura sauce ■ Grated diakon and ginger ■ Tempura

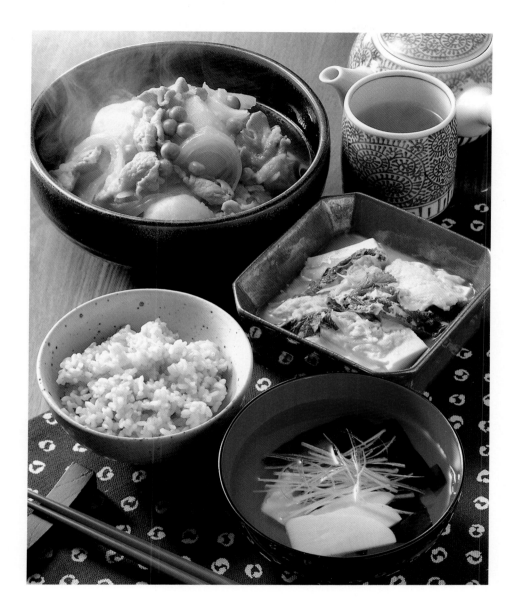

DAY ONE DINNER: Pork and Potatoes ■ Tofu and diakon leaves ■ Rice ■ Wakame soup

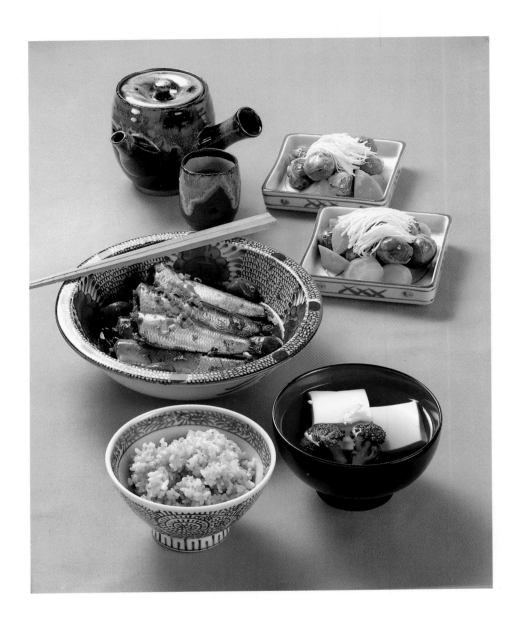

DAY TWO DINNER: Brussel sprout and carrot salads ■
Sardines in umeboshi sauce ■ Rice ■ Broccoli and tofu soup

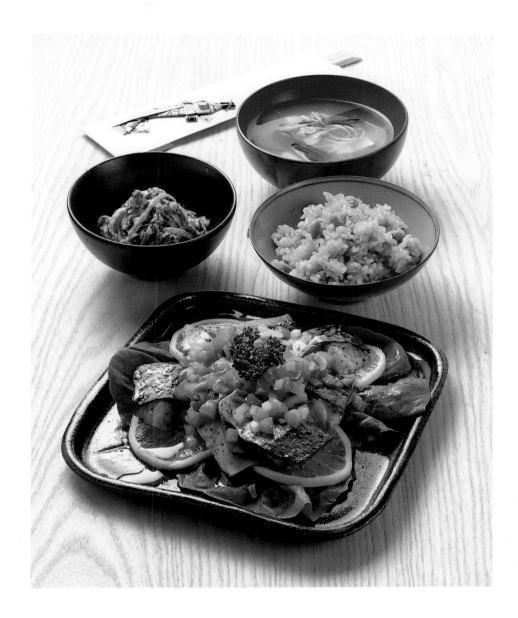

DAY THREE LUNCH: Wakame and tofu miso soup ■ Tofu and vegetable mix ■ Rice ■ Mackeral with tomato and onion dressing

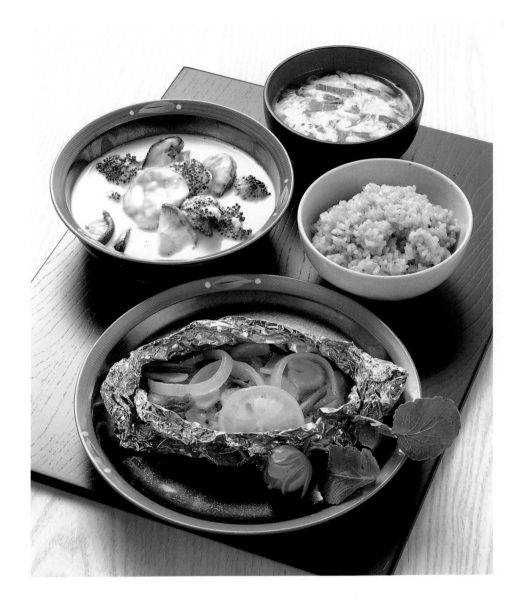

DAY THREE DINNER: Egg and leek soup ■ Creamed broccoli and mushrooms ■ Rice ■ Steamed chicken

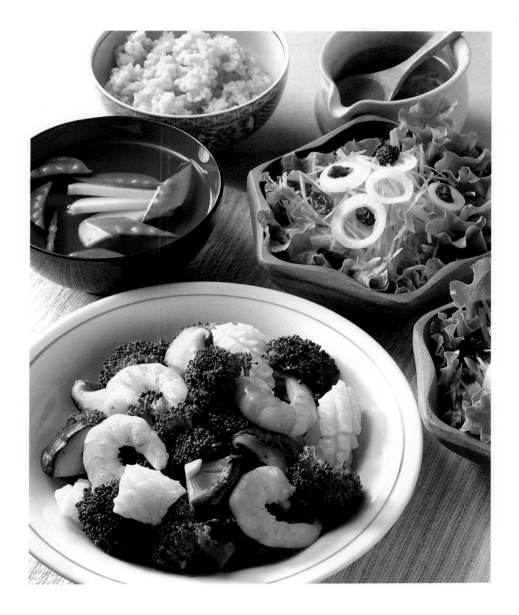

DAY FIVE LUNCH: Rice ■ Clear soup (with kamaboko and snow peas) ■ Salad dressing ■ Carrot salad ■ Squid, shrimp and broccoli

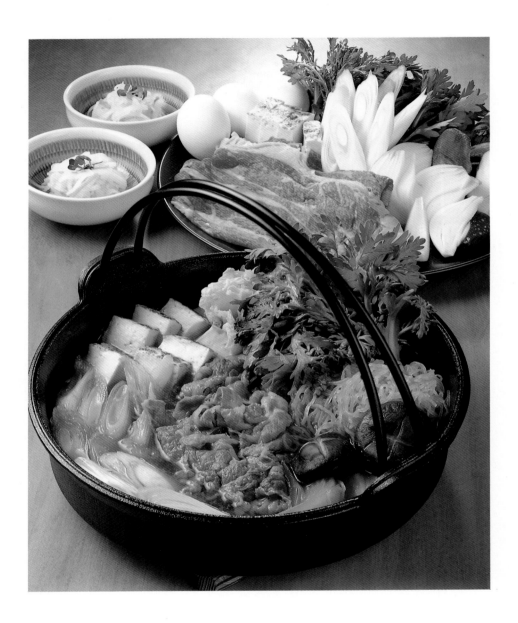

DAY FIVE DINNER: Vinegared daikon and carrots ■ Sukiyaki
ingredients ■ Sukiyaki

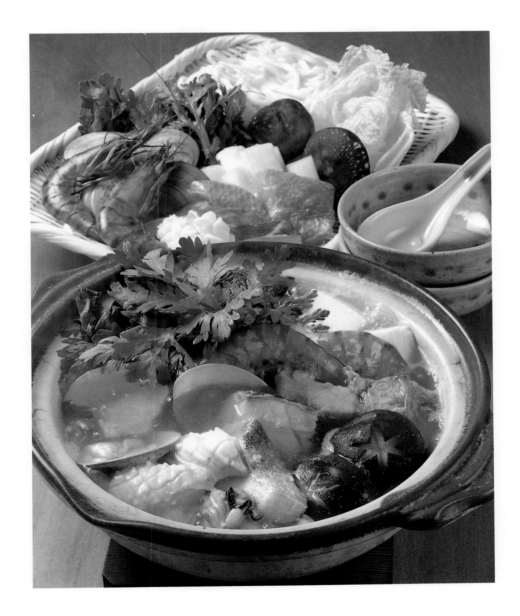

DAY SEVEN DINNER: Fish casserole ingredients ■ Fish casserole

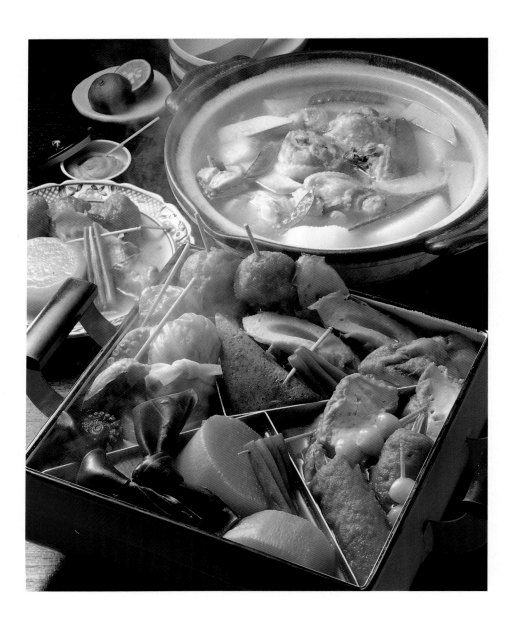

CASSEROLES: Chicken mizutaki (top) ■ Oden (bottom)

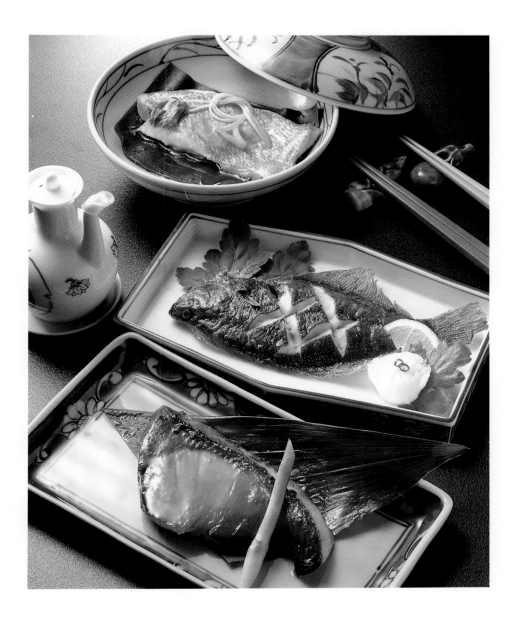

FISH DISHES: Steamed sea bream and kombu (top) ■ Deep fried flatfish (middle) ■ Yellowtail teriyaki (bottom)

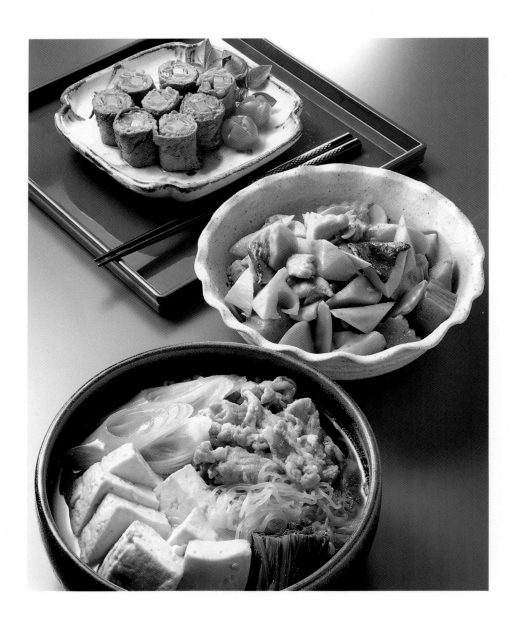

MEAT DISHES: Rolled beef ■ Boiled chicken mixed with vegetables ■ Pork and tofu

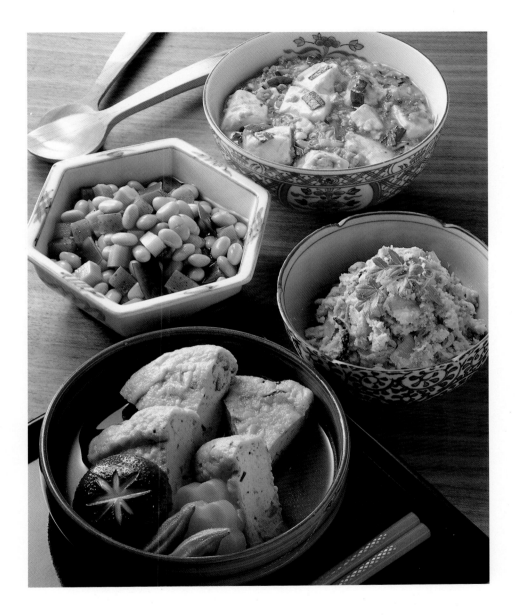

BEAN AND TOFU DISHES: Mabadofu ■ Boiled beans with mushrooms and carrots ■ Okara ■ Gammodoki, shiitake and vegetables

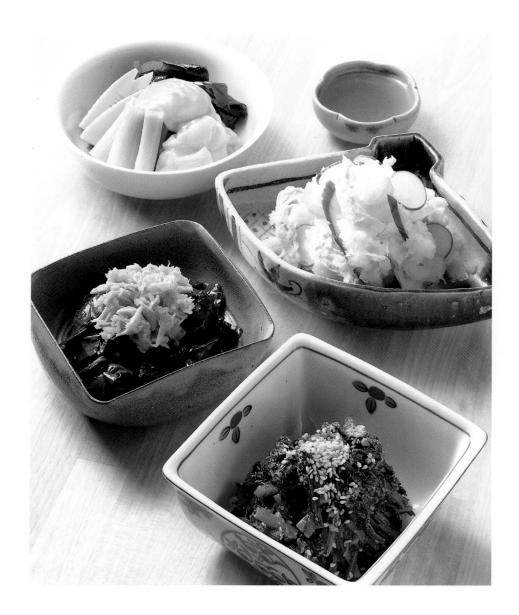

Clams and vegetables with mustard/vinegar and miso
dressing ■ Salad dressing ■ Spinach and tuna salad ■
Shungiku with sesame seeds

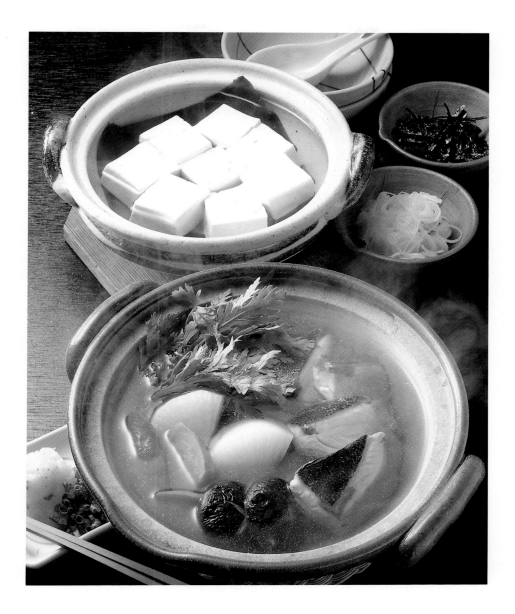

Boiled tofu and kombu ■ Nori ■ Sliced daikon ■ Yellowtail nabe

Ingredients

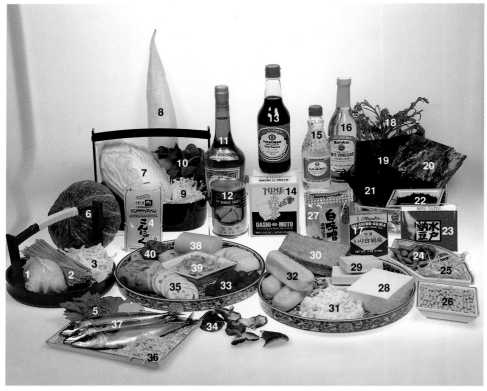

1. shiratake	13. soy sauce	27. miso
2. soba	14. dashino moto	28. tofu
3. udon	15. mirin	29. koya-dofu
4. konnyaku	16. rice vinegar	30. atsuage
5. shiso	17. sesame seeds	31. okara
6. japanese pumpkin (kabocha)	18. shungiku	32. aburage
	19. nori	33. umeboshi
7. hakusai	20. konbu	34. shiitake
8. daikon	21. wakame	35. lotus root
9. enokitake mushrooms	22. hijiki	36. shirasuboshi
10. trefoil (mitsuba)	23. natto	37. saba
11. sake	24. edamame	38. kamaboko
12. bamboo shoots (takenoko)	25. soybean sprouts	39. katsuobushi
	26. daizu	40. gammodoki

Chapter 7

How The Very Old Live and Eat

If you want to live to a ripe and healthy old age, avoid needless worry and stress and don't eat too much.

Japanese who have lived to be 100 years old lead happy and alert lives. It's not that they are fully satisfied with their lives. They all have hopes and unfulfilled desires. Izumi, the 120-year-old, had always hoped to tear down his house and build a better one before he died.

Another thing to keep in mind is that the diet of these oldsters hardly ever exceeded 1,800 calories per day.

The life of Mr. Izumi was a typical example of how many elderly live in Japan. The staple in his diet was sweet potatoes. The other foods he ate consisted of vegetables, seaweed, tofu, fish, pork, chicken and eggs. All the vegetable he ate were grown by himself and included spinach, mustard leaf, peas with the pods and pumpkin. He also caught all the fish he ate which were mackerel, sardines, flying fish and others. He also liked shell fish, and when the season was right, would hunt abalone in the shallows. He kept chickens and often ate eggs. Izumi also enjoyed chicken and pork on those rare occasions when it was available.

The oldster's diet also included "recreational foods." Among them were sugar cane which grew near his home. He also often ate brown sugar, but absolutely avoided refined sugar.

Alcohol was another of Izumi's pleasures. He drank a glass daily of shochu (a spirit made from brown sugar) daily. That fact caused a boom of daily shochu drinking and large profits for shochu makers, especially the manufacturer of the brand that Izumi drank.

However, the common thread linking the diet of Japan's oldsters is that they all eat protein daily and consume milk and eggs — items that some Western dieticians frown upon for the elderly. Additionally, they all eat fish, pork, beef and poultry plus tofu and miso.

There is an important factor in the consumption of protein by the elderly — it is that protein makes up just under 20 percent of the total calories. This is rather high when compared to levels recommended by Western nutritionists, but on the other hand, fat intakes measured only 16.1 percent of total calories with the remaining calories coming from carbohydrates.

Whether this level of protein intake is ideal or not cannot be easily determined. What is certain is that reducing the amount, even for short periods, can be fatal. There have been a number of medically observed cases where this has happened. They quickly display all the symptoms of protein deficiency: high serum urea levels and water retention in the abdominal cavity.

However, this high level of protein intake must be considered in the context of total calories consumed daily. The centenarians studied in Okinawa average 13.6 calories per pound of bodyweight.

That is a very low level and means that a 110 lbs. woman should eat only 1,500 calories daily while a 170 lbs. man should have around 2,300 calories. Remember, however, that these elderly persons are lean and fit. They have low bodyfat and maintain ideal bodyweight. From this, we can deduce that one secret to a long and healthy life is to set the number of calories we need based on how much we weigh.

Another factor found in the diets of those 100 years and older is the high amounts of dark-green vegetables and seaweed such as kombu and wakame.

And, as far as salt intake, the centenarians of Okinawa don't worry about this. Still, they consume less than the average Japanese. Obviously, since food intake is lower, salt intake is also proportionately lower. Miso soup is usually taken at least once daily and this provides at least one gram of salt. Needless to say, there are no salt shakers on the table, so salt is never added once the food is served on the table.

Let's look   at some typical daily menus of Okinawa's 100 year oldsters.

Example 1. Mr. Goto, 102 years old

BREAKFAST

A glass of milk

Three slices of whole wheat bread
   (no butter or jams are added)

LUNCH

One bowl of rice

A bowl of miso soup

Wakame: bean sprouts

One egg

Tofu mixed with dark-green vegetables and shell fish

DINNER

One bowl of rice

Beef soup

Liver

Dark green vegetable

Potato

Example 2. Mrs. Kureha; 101 years old

BREAKFAST

A half glass of milk

Sweet potato

LUNCH

A half a bowl of rice gruel (okayu)

A bowl of miso soup

Wakame

Noodles

One boiled egg

One banana

A half glass of orange juice

DINNER

A half bowl of rice gruel (okayu)

A bowl of boiled pork, kombu, and daikon

Snack

One banana

Example 3. Mrs. Kukita, 103 years old

BREAKFAST

One bowl of rice

One bowl of miso soup

One egg

Chinese cabbage

LUNCH

One bowl of rice

One bowl of miso soup

One egg

Cucumber

Fish with dark green vegetables

DINNER

One bowl of rice

A bowl of boiled meat, dark green vegetables and tofu

■

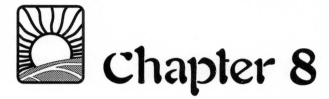

Chapter 8

A Common Sense Approach To Exercise and Longevity

Man is the only animal that engages in exercise just for the sake of exercise, sometimes forcing himself to the limit of his physical ability.

It is an artificial activity resulting from the sedentary life of an office job where the only physical activity may be getting up from our computer desk to have lunch or something to drink.

To avoid the harmful results of that lifestyle, millions of Americans have gone on an exercise boom. They are jogging, participating in aerobics or buying stationary bicycles or rowing machines that will allow them to exercise to their heart's delight.

However, it is a fallacy to believe that exercise will add years to your life. Many who verge on fanaticism about exercise may face just the opposite result and die young.

Exercise and Life Span

Not one of the centenarians studied at my institute ever intensely trained for any sport or excercised vigorously for any sustained period of time. Yet, these 100 year olds were not sedentary, they were moderately active, moving around and completing daily chores. Their lives can best be described as "easy going."

We can deduce from this that a high level of activity throughout life is a negative factor in reaching extreme old age. The three common factors found among these centenarians is that they eat a low-calorie, nutritionally balanced diet, are only moderately active and cheerful and optimistic.

Research also clearly shows a relationship between longevity and exercise. One lab experiment with rats showed that sedentary rats who overeat have a 25 percent shorter life span than rats which overeat and exercise. Rats which undereat and exercise have a 20 percent greater life expectancy than the overeating but exercising rats. However, those rats which undereat and are sedentary live 25 percent longer than the exercising, undereating rats.

The conclusion is inevitable: high intensity exercise can shorten your life.

Cardiovascular Fitness and Exercise

Marathon runners have always been upheld as examples of healthy and superbly fit athletes.

Yet, just the opposite may be true. During the 1960 Olympics in Rome, 89 marathon runners were given electro-cardiograms. The results were disturbing. More than 77 per cent of these distance runners registered abnormal heart rhythms. While these abnormalities may not have been life threatening or an impediment to performance, their long term implications and effect on longevity are cause for concern.

Many athletes have irregular heart beats, called arrhythmias. Even healthy people develop this condition under stress and intense athletic training (such as training for a marathon) involves extremely stressful activity. Subjecting yourself to such stress for long periods in your life may be unwise if you hope to be healthy through your old age.

Take for example what happens when your body is under stress. It produces cortisol, and the longer and more serious the stress, the more cortisol is produced. That substance suppresses the production of interferon, a major chemical needed for the body's immune response to fight viral infections. The inhibition of interferon production may be one reason that both animals and people who are under constant stress develop diseases such as cancer at a higher than expected rate.

While these remarks are speculative, you must consider them carefully before engaging in strenuous and intense exercise.

It's not that we oppose exericse. It's ideal for those who lead sedentary lives such as working in offices. An exercise program may be necessary for improved health. What we caution against is excessive exercise which, like overeating, can shorten your life.

There appears to be an optimum level for exercise intensity and constantly exceeding this level could negatively effect your life span. Determining this level is not simple.

Exercise Intensity – The Ideal Level

There is no set way to determine the exercise-intensity level for everyone. Each person has a different endurance limit achieved through training. Some physiologists maintain that 15 miles of jogging per week is ideal for cardiovascular fitness, but more than that is detrimental. That may be true for the general population, but it should not be blindly followed. Some people may be genetically capable of intense training without suffering harmful effects, while others can be harmed by a very moderate exercise program.

If you've decided to exercise, determine you own level of intensity by "listening" to your body. Follow this general rule: push yourself only to the point that you become moderately tired.

Age is a major consideration when you start an exercise program. Research shows that exercise is beneficial when done throughout an animals' life. However, when exercise is started after middle age, it will shorten the expected life span.

Who Should Exercise?

Some people do not need exercise. If you do lots of walking or lead an active life, it could be that your level of activity is ideal and adding an exercise regimen may actually shorten your life, especially if you are not particularly interested in exercising. Additionally, there are some people who just are not constitutionally suited to exercise. These people are just not athletic, but may otherwise be perfectly healthy. It's up to you to determine which type you are.

On the other hand, there are those who can definitely benefit from exercise: those who lead an inactive life and eat more calories than they use in their daily activities. Research shows that if you are dieting to lose weight, exercise will help you.

Common Sense Rules for Exercising

START OUT SLOWLY

Never plunge into an exercise program by going fullout the first day. Obviously, if you are starting an exercise program it is common sense to consider yourself out of shape. So, start out slowly, gradually increasing the level of intensity. Don't try completing a workout someone has given you the first time you try it. Work up gradually to the required intensity.

EXERCISE REGULARLY

Once you have decided to begin exercising, stick with it and make it part of your daily schedule. Don't be fanatical about it though. If you are even mildly ill, don't exercise. If you are busy with work, skip exercising because all it will do is add stress.

Avoid exercising hard one week, skipping one week, then trying to pick up at the same level a week later. That type of schedule can hurt you more than help you.

RECUPERATION

Recuperation is important to any exercise program. Some athletes, who train constantly at high levels, develop symptoms that include swollen glands, constant tiredness, insomnia or increased sleep requirements, loss of appetite, and weight loss.

There are no studies which have related overtraining to longevity, but common sense alone would indicate that excessive exercise shortens your potential for a long life.

Try to follow this schedule: exercise only every other day, or even every three days if the exercise is intense. Skipping days allows your body a chance to recover from the stress caused by exercising. However, if you decide to exercise every day, alternate with days of low intensity with days of high intensity. Keep in mind, that the older you are, the longer it will take you to recuperate.

Recuperation is also affected by the intensity of exercise. Exercising before you have fully recuperated leads to over-training. For some athletes recuperation time is impossible. Marathon runners, for example, must train at extremely high levels to build up endurance. This continuous high level of training may be so intense that these athletes simply do not have time to recuperate.

What's the Best Kind of Exercise?

Carefully consider these points when deciding what type of exercise or exercises you are going to perform.

CONVENIENCE

Walking is the most convenient exercise and is something you can fit into your regular daily activities, it's also the safest of all exercises. Skip elevators and instead use the stairs. Walk to the store instead of driving. Swimming is also an excellent activity if a pool is available.

THE EXERCISE SHOULD NOT CAUSE INJURIES

Avoid exercising to the point where it can cause injuries. This can only defeat the main objective of exercising which is to promote health and, thereby, longevity. There is nothing wrong with jogging or other aerobic exercises, which are excellent for promoting cardiovascular fitness, just don't overdo them. Exercising to intensely can painfully injure tendons and joints in your legs. Some people are prone to this type of injury. Make sure, before you start, that your body is not prone to this type of weakness.

Injuries can also result from participating in sports which require quick reflexes. These involve sudden movements that place severe stress on joints, muscles and tendons. Avoid these injuries by warming up before you start competing. Secondly, strengthen all the muscles and tendons in your body by some form of weight or resistance training.

WARMING UP AND STRETCHING

Warming up is critical to avoiding injuries and making sure your muscles will achieve their peak performance. Many injuries are caused by failure to warm up properly. Don't think that this just means raising your heartbeat and breathing hard. It means warming up those particular muscles that will be used in your particular exercise, whether it be jogging, swimming, tennis or racquet ball.

Another major point to remember is never stretch cold muscles. That type of activity can easily cause microinjuries which can become aggravated when you start the strenuous part of your training. Remember that stretching is something you do after completing your exercise session. It is an important adjunct to exercises in which the full use of the muscle is not used, such as jogging.

Keep in mind that different people have different stretching abilities. Some have very flexible bodies with a remarkable range of motion. Others lack that flexibility and no matter how hard they try they will never attain the range of motion of more flexible people. Stretching exercises can increase your range of motion, but don't blindly follow a coach or trainer who insists you become as flexible as rubber. Deliberately and slowly find your own limits.

■

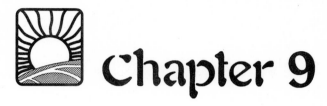

Chapter 9

How to Cook

Way back in caveman times, the cave chef was limited in what he or she could prepare. Raw was the rage then. You dragged something in, ripped away the hairy stuff, squatted around the cave entrance and enjoyed an outdoor meal.

Then, someone discovered fire and that raw stuff tasted better if it was thrown into the flames. Barbecue was in.

Still later, the best of the cave chefs invented pots. They found that if you boiled water and tossed in chunks of plants or animals, minus the hairy stuff, it sometimes tasted good. This greatly expanded the daily menus. The great cave chefs went wild. They gathered all sorts of plants, tossed them in boiling pots and picked their teeth while they waited to see what would come out. Most was nauseating and was dumped out. Some however, was tasty.

So began modern cooking.

After thousands of years, we have learned that the way you cook your foods affects your health, just as much as the kind of foods you eat.

Some foods are best eaten raw, others must be cooked to make them edible and still others must be cooked in a certain way or else they may not be good for you.

In Japan, many foods are eaten raw, including fish — a practice that has spread to the United States where many Americans now eat sushi (thin slices of raw fish wrapped in rice).

I believe that many foods would be better if they were eaten raw rather than cooked. Cooking destroys some of their nutrients and the digestive enzymes they contain.

However, some foods need to be cooked at high temperatures since this is the only way harmful substances can be neutralized. For example, some dark green vegetables, if eaten raw, contain unhealthy substances that bind with iron and other minerals in our body. Cooking eliminates these substances. Japanese occasionally eat raw eggs, but cooking them is healthier.

The best method of making food edible is by boiling, even though some water-soluble vitamins are lost (boiling in large pieces, minimizes this loss). Steam cooking is another method similar to boiling. Additionally, many dishes are prepared by wrapping them in aluminum foil and steaming or baking them.

A very unhealthy way to prepare fish or meats is to roast them over an open flame. When flames singe meat a number of cancer causing substances are created. One of them is benzo[a]pyrene, a substance so carcinogenic that when it is applied to the skin of mice it causes cancer within 24 hours. This substance is also carried in tobacco smoke, one reason why lung cancer among smokers is so high. This method of cooking is used widely in northern Japan where cancer in the abdominal area is widespread.

Using a microwave oven is probably the safest way to cook foods since vitamin loss is very low.

Vegetable Oils Can be Unhealthy

Never leave vegetable oils sitting on a shelf. They should always be refrigerated soon after opening to avoid becoming rancid.

Rancidity occurs whether the oil is a saturated or unsaturated fat. The rancidity begins when the oil or fat container is exposed to oxygen which alters certain substances in the oils. Once inside the body, these subtances burst cell membrances and attack the DNA inside. If DNA is eventually altered, cells go wild and produce cancer.

Saturated fats, however, are chemically more stable than unsaturated fats, so they turn rancid at a much slower rate. The big danger is with unsaturated vegetable oils.

Whenever you first open a bottle or can of vegetable oil, the oil is of good quality. These oils also have additives or natural substances such as vitamin E, that keep the oils fresh for long periods. However, when first exposed to oxygen the deterioration of its quality begins. Take a look at Graph 11 which shows the difference in the rate of deterioration between cooking oils that have no additives and those with vitamin E. Remember, that some rancidity develops within the first three or four days after a container of oil is opened and not refrigerated. It is not enough to be smelled, but nevertheless it is still there.

Reputable manufacturers of cooking oil are meticulous in making sure that their product is in perfect condition when it reaches the kitchen. The problem is sometimes in buying oil in large amounts. It may save pennies, but it could shorten your life.

Consider this long term study involving middle-aged men to determine the effect of a low-fat diet on the incidence of cardio-vascular disease. One group ate a diet high in saturated animal fats, such as mlk, eggs, butter, and cheese. The other group's diet was low in these fats, but high in unsaturated fats found in vegetable oils.

The results shocked the medical researchers. They discovered that while the number of cardio-vascular disease was low among the group whose diet was low in saturated fats but high in unsaturated fats, the number of cancer cases had soared far higher than expected. Was it possible that animal fat provided protection against cancer? The answer was just the reverse: it was the vegetable oils that were causing the cancer.

Yet, unsaturated fats found in vegetable oils are essential to health. Your body cannot make them from the food you eat. Moreover, the fatty acids in vegetable oils lower the cholesterol levels in your blood and are important for maintaining healthy and beautiful skin.

A few tips allows you to maintain these positive factors while avoiding the pitfalls of rancid oil. Keep them in mind the next time you buy cooking oil.

■ Buy oils in small containers and use them quickly after opening. Remember, even when oil contains additives to keep it fresh, it is still becoming rancid.

■ Never store oils at room temperature for long periods of time. In fact, if you are not going to use the oil right away, store it in the refrigerator. The oil will solidify, but it will remain fresh longer than if you had kept it at room temperature. Generally, oil should never be stored at more than 10 degrees of its melting point.

■ Light also speeds up the chemical reaction that causes rancidity, so store oil in dark, cool places, in tightly sealed containers.

■ Throw away oil that has been used for deep-frying foods. Oils that have been heated to high temperatures become unstable and deteriorate more quickly. The high temperature also destroys vitamin E, a natural occurring preservative. Use fresh oil when you fry tempura.

■ Never eat fried foods that have been standing around. This includes tempura and snack foods, such as potato chips. Foods cooked in oil and with large surface areas become rancid very quickly. Margarine, biscuits and chocolate bars, which are high in oil content, are examples of other foods that you should show caution after opening them.

■ Reputable manufacturers generally follow strict policy in the quality of their preparation and packaging of foods, but once the finished product is distributed to wholesalers and retailers, storage conditions may not be ideal. Packaged foods usually have a shelf life of about nine months, so always check the manufacturing date. If it was produced too long ago, don't buy it.

■ Smoked fish and meats and sun-dried fish and meats are also unhealthy. The fats and oils in the meat and fish will certainly become rancid in these curing processes. Eat only fresh fish and meat.

When in doubt, throw it out. That is a good rule to follow if you have questions about a food product. The best way to be sure that the food you eat is safe, is to prepare it in your home. In the last several years, Japanese foods, such as sushi, tempura, and tofu, have become quite popular as health foods. However, these are served mainly in restaurants where they may not be fresh. You can guarantee that freshness by learning how to prepare these dishes at home and at the same time discover why Japanese foods are so wonderful.

■

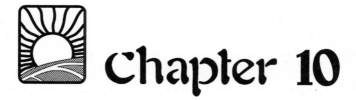

Chapter 10

The Japanese Supernutrition Food Ingredients

To start your supernutrition diet you will have to buy the necessary foods. This chapter lists those items which are available at any supermarket or Oriental food store.

Vegetables

Bamboo shoots — These are found in many Japanese dishes and often are part of boiled or stir-fried mixed vegetables.

Chinese Cabbage — This vegetable is used mainly in one-pot dishes such as sukiyaki or stir-fried vegetables. It is also called "Napa cabbage," or just "Napa."

Enokitake Mushrooms — These crisp and aromatic mushrooms are a common ingredient in soups and sukiyaki.

Japanese pumpkin — Japanese pumpkin is not the orange type used during Halloween. It is green and similar to squash.

Japanese radish — (Daikon) a white radish about 18 inches long.

Konnyaku — Konnyaku is a jellied paste, with a high calcium content made from a tuberous root called devil's tongue.

It is usually sold in three-inch square blocks and consists of about 97 percent water. While tasteless, it absorbs the flavor of other foods.

Lotus Root — Long used as a folk medicine in Japan, lotus roots have a crisp texture and are excellent when boiled with other vegetables like carrots and kelp.

Shiitake — A popular mushroom in Japan considered to have medicinal properties. Contains substances that inhibit malignant tumors and lowers blood cholesterol.

Shirataki — Konnyaku in long thin strips. Often served with beef dishes like sukiyaki.

Shiso — A mint-like leaf from the beefsteak plant. Used as a garnish in many Japanese dishes and to accompany raw fish and tempura.

Shungiku — (Chrysanthemum Leaves) — These leaves are boiled like spinach and is the standard vegetable (along with Chinese cabbage) used in sukiyaki. The leaves are high in calcium and vitamin A. Don't overcook them. These are not the leaf of the commonly grown flower.

Trefoil (mitsuba) — Green leaves used as a garnish.

Yuzu — A small citrus fruit, the peels of which are used as a garnish in many Japanese soups.

Seaweeds

Kelp (Kombu) — The basic ingredient for making soup stock. It is also used in many one-pot dishes. Kombu has a natural white covering which should not be washed off. Instead wipe it with a damp towel then soak it in lukewarm water until it increases to about twice its original size.

Hijiki —This has the highest calcium content of all seaweeds and is also high in iron. A serving of 50 grams will supply you with more than 100 percent of your daily calcium and iron requirements. Often served in a small dish with carrot slivers or peas.

Nori — Also known as "laver." Best known in the West for use in making sushi. Extremely high in vitamins and minerals.

Wakame — Ideal for salads and clear Japanese soups. The salt can be removed by soaking in cold water. Before using, it should be soaked in warm water until it doubles in size.

Soybeans and Soybean Products

Fresh green soybeans (edamame) — Fresh soybeans boiled with the pods.

Soybean sprouts

Dried soybeans — Mature dried soybeans are available packaged throughout the U.S.

Tofu — Tofu (bean curd) — comes in two main varieties: cotton (or firm) tofu and silk (soft) tofu.

Deep-fried tofu cutlets (atsuage) — Cakes of tofu, deep fried.

Deep-fried tofu puffs (aburage) — Puffs of tofu, deep fried.

Gammadoki — Deep-fried tofu patties with thinly-diced vegetables, sesame seeds, and seaweed.

Freeze-dried tofu — Frozen and dried tofu cakes.

Grilled Tofu — Pressed and grilled tofu.

Okara — The residue of crushed soybeans which have been used to make tofu.

Miso-Fermented soybean paste. — There are two types: white miso, which is actually yellow, and red miso, which is brown. White miso has the lowest salt content. Besides being used for soup, it is also used as a dressing.

Natto — Whole fermented soybeans. Popular for breakfast. Often eaten together with rice for breakfast.

Noodles

Soba — Long brown, thin noodles made from buckwheat flour mixed with unbleached flour. The amount of buckwheat in soba ranges from 40 percent to 100 percent.

Udon — Thick, round, white noodles made of flour.

Condiments

Bonito flakes — Made from the shavings of dried bonito fish. and used as a base for soup stocks or as a garnish with boiled vegetables.

Mirin — A sweet syrupy rice wine (sake) used in many Japanese dishes.

Sake — Japan's traditional "wine." It is made from steamed rice and a yeast called koji. Although it is mainly an alcoholic beverage, it is also a major ingredient in many Japanese dishes.

Sesame seeds — Sesame seeds (goma) are used as a garnish in many Japanese dishes. For the best use of its nutrients, they should be toasted and then ground. They come in two varieties, white and black seeds. Both are extremely high in calcium and magnesium.

Soy sauce — The main seasoning used in Japanese foods. A must when eating sushi. Although high in salt, a low-salt soy sauce is available.

Rice Vinegar — Sweeter than western vinegar. Made from white rice. It softens hard vegetables during cooking.

Wasabi — Japanese horseradish. An extremely sharp tasting green paste used on sushi and other dishes.

■

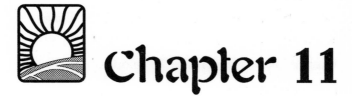

Chapter 11

A One-Week Supernutrition Menu

The following menus are typical of meals served in Japanese homes. Many follow the traditional meal structure but also contain casserole dishes plus Western-style breakfasts which have become popular over the past 40 years.

These menus include items selected from all the four food groups and are low in saturated fats since meat and fish are limited to no more than 200 grams a day, ensuring an adequate but not excessive protein intake.

We recommend you use brown rice and whole grain bread, providing you with adequate fiber plus vitamin E which is removed from white rice and refined flour.

The calories in these meals may be a bit low for Americans, who have larger physiques on average than Japanese. The average American should probably increase the portions and add healthy snacks to bring the calories up to 1,800 to 2,000 a day.

DAY ONE MENU

BREAKFAST

Fruit yogurt (8 oz.) = 120 calories

Omelete (two eggs, 1 oz. cheese) = 215 calories

Buttered toast = 105 calories

Orange juice (6 oz glass) = 75 calories

Total calories = 515

LUNCH

Miso soup = 30 calories

Tempura = 196 calories

Hijiki and sesame seed salad = 80 calories

Rice = 160 calories

Total calories = 466

DINNER

Wakame soup = 19 calories

Pork and potatoes = 253 calories

Tofu with diakon leaves = 155 calories

Rice = 160 calories

Total calories = 587

Total Day One Calories = 1,547

DAY TWO MENU

BREAKFAST

Pizza toast = 230 calories

Fruit = 80 calories

Eggs (two) boiled or poached = 160 calories

Total calories = 425

LUNCH

Miso soup = 30 calories

Beef, shirataki and tofu = 226 calories

Daikon salad = 30 calories

Rice = 160 calories

Total calories = 446

DINNER

Broccoli and tofu soup = 36 calories

Sardines in umeboshi sauce = 258 calories

Brussel sprouts and carrot salad = 52 calories

Rice = 160 calories

Total calories = 506

Total Day Two Calories = 1,437

DAY THREE MENU

BREAKFAST

Frozen yogurt and fruit = 200 calories

Boiled beans with mushrooms and carrots = 147 calories

Boiled spinach and bean sprouts = 26 calories

Rice = 160 calories

Total calories = 534

LUNCH

Wakame and tofu miso soup = 66 calories

Mackeral with tomato and onion dressing = 267 calories

Tofu and vegetable mix = 95 calories

Rice = 160 calories

Total calories = 588

DINNER

Egg and leek soup = 43 calories

Steamed chicken = 194 calories

Creamed Broccoli and Mushrooms = 252 calories

Rice = 160 calories

Total calories = 649

Total Day Three calories = 1,771

DAY FOUR MENU

BREAKFAST

Yellowtail Nabe = 300 calories

Rice = 160 calories

Total calories = 460

LUNCH

Red snapper soup = 58 calories

Mabodofu = 137 calories

Spinach and tuna salad = 52 calories

Rice = 160 calories

Total calories = 407

DINNER

Miso soup = 30 calories

Chicken and cashew nuts = 243 calories

Stir-fried corn, peas, and cheese = 174 calories

Rice = 160 calories

Total calories = 607

Total Day Four Calories = 1,474

DAY FIVE MENU

BREAKFAST

Toast and butter = 210 calories

Lowfat milk or yogurt (8 oz) = 120 calories

Fruit = 80 calories

Total calories = 410

LUNCH

Clear soup = 30 calories

Shrimp, squid and broccoli = 53 calories

Carrot salad = 73 calories

Rice = 160 calories

Total calories = 316

DINNER

Miso soup = 30 calories

Sukiyaki = 524 calories

Vinegared daikon and carrots = 34 calories

Raw egg = 80 calories

Rice = 160 calories

Total calories = 828

Total Day Five Calories = 1,594

DAY SIX MENU

BREAKFAST

Two slices toast and butter = 210 calories

Egg-cheese omelet = 335 calories

Total calories = 545

LUNCH

Miso soup = 30 calories

Pork and sweet potatoes = 148 calories

Daikon, carrots and cucumber salad = 25 calories

Rice = 160 calories

Total calories = 363 calories

DINNER

Miso soup = 30 calories

Salmon saute = 248 calories

Spinach and bean sprouts sautéed = 40 calories

Rice = 160 calories

Total calories = 478

Total Day Four calories = 1,386

DAY SEVEN MENU

BREAKFAST

Fruit and yogurt = 200 calories

Gammodoki, shiitake and vegetables = 130 calories

Rice = 160 calories

Total calories = 491

LUNCH

Egg and Leek soup = 43 calories

Chicken and Chinese cabbage (Hakusai or Napa) = 130 calories

Okara = 122 calories

Rice = 160 calories

Total calories = 455 calories

DINNER

Fish casserole = 284 calories

Udon = 160 calories

Total calories = 444

Total Day Seven Calories = 1,390

■

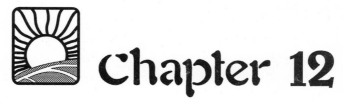

Chapter 12

Soups

The most important thing you have to consider in cooking Japanese is the preparation of the stock, called dashi in Japanese. The most common ingredient in all Japanese stock is the seaweed kombu. You can make stock with kelp alone or together with either dried bonito flakes or dried sardines

In Japan, most households depend on packaged stock, a time-saving convenience in which excellent products are used. However, if you have the time you might want to make stock to ensure that you get all the nutrients from the kelp and other items that are used.

Making Stock with Kelp

Use a 6-inch strip of dried kelp. When you remove it from the package use a damp cloth to wipe off the white substance covering it. Soak the kelp in four cups of water for about an hour then heat the water. Remove the kelp as soon as the water boils and let it cool.

Making Stock with Kelp and Bonito Flakes.

Basic stock (used for clear soups)

Follow the recipe above for making stock, then add 1/4 cup of water and heat. As the stock begins to boil, add one cup of bonito flakes. As it boils, it will foam. At this point, lower the flame and simmer for 10 seconds. Remove from heat and add a pinch of salt. The bonito flakes will sink. Strain immediately. The stock is ready for use.

Secondary Stock (used for thick soups and cooking oden)

Use the kelp and bonito flakes remaining from making basic stock. Add four cups of water and heat. When it begins to boil, lower the flame and simmer for 15 minutes then strain and store for use.

Making Stock with Dried Sardines (usually for miso soups)

Wash and soak about 10 dried sardines in five cups of water for up to three hours (the longer you soak them, the stronger the stock). Heat to about 100 degrees fahrenheit and then strain.

Miso Soups and Clear Soups

The traditional Japanese diet includes two main kinds of soup: miso (misoshiru) and clear soups (suimono). These soups can be made in a number of variations by altering the ingredients, but the base remains the same. Miso soups are made using a soup stock and miso. Clear soups use only basic stock.

Different kinds of soups can be made by adding two or more types of vegetables, or a vegetable and fish or tofu. Below are examples of a miso soup and a clear soup.

TOFU AND WAKAME MISO SOUP (serves four)

Ingredients

4 cups of stock

5 tbs of miso

1 pack of tofu

1/3 ounce of dried wakame

Directions

Boil the stock and add the tofu and wakame. Place the miso in a mixing bowl and add a bit of the boiling stock and stir until it has dissolved. Pour into soup and allow it to boil momentarily. Remove from heat and serve.

BROCCOLI AND TOFU SOUP (serves four)

Ingredients

1 head of broccoli

100 grams (1/2 cake) of soft tofu

3 cups of soup stock

1/2 tsp of salt

2 tsp of soy sauce

Lemon peels

Directions

Cut the broccoli into bite-size pieces and cut the tofu into two-inch squares. Boil the broccoli in water with a pinch of salt. In a sauce pan put three cups of soup stock and add the boiled broccoli and tofu and heat. Add the salt and soy sauce. When the tofu is done, remove from heat and serve. Sprinkle lemon peels over soup just before serving.

Here are some other combinations you can use for soups, both miso and clear: bamboo shoots and wakame; clams and shiitake; chicken and a vegetable or a seaweed; white fish and scallions.

In the following recipes you will find variations of both these kinds of soup. You may also want to experiment with combinations of your own.

Rice Dishes

How to Cook Rice

If you're going to prepare rice on a daily basis, the best time saver is an automatic rice cooker. These little gadgets prepare rice perfectly every time and provide marks indicating the exact proportion of rice to water. Automatic rice cookers are available at most Oriental food stores.

In Japan, rice is served by itself in a bowl and is eaten with the other dishes. However, many ingredients can be added to the rice. For example, small dried fish, bonito flakes or natto are some of the items you can add to the rice.

Two such rice dishes are rice porridge (zosui) and rice with bamboo shoots (takenoko gohan).

RICE AND CRAB/VEGETABLE PORRIDGE (serves four)

This is the Japanese hangover cure or for someone who might not be feeling well. You can change the ingredients to suit your taste or use whatever is available.

Ingredients

3 cups of cooked rice

4 cups of soup stock

1 cake of soft tofu

4 ounces of crab sticks

1 bunch of trefoil (mitsuba)

2 whipped eggs

a dash of salt

2 tsp of sake

Directions

Cut tofu into bite-size pieces, the crab sticks into 1 1/4 inch lengths and the trefoil (mitsuba) into 1 inch lengths.

Place the rice and soup stock in a covered pot then place over a high flame. As soon as it boils, remove the cover, reduce to a low flame and add tofu and crab sticks. Allow it to boil again and then add sake and salt, and stir. Pour in the whipped eggs and trefoil while stirring. Remove from heat, replace lid and steam until the eggs are done.

RICE WITH BAMBOO SHOOTS (serves four)

Ingredients

3 cups of cooked rice

7 ounces of boiled bamboo shoots

1/2 cup of sake

1 tbs of light soy sauce

2 tsp of mirin

1/2 tsp of salt

an appropriate quantity of trefoil stems

Directions

Thoroughly wash rice and let it stand for about 30 minutes. Cut the bamboo shoots into thin bite-sized pieces and soak in the mixture of mirin, light soy sauce and salt. Briefly boil the trefoil stems. In a suitable pot, combine 3.3 cups of water with the rice, bamboo shoots and the mixture in which the shoots have soaked. Stir. When the bamboo shoots rise to the surface, boil briefly, remove from heat and serve. Sprinkle the trefoil stems on top just before serving.

BOILED GREEN VEGETABLES (Ohitashi)

Spinach and Bonito Flakes

Ingredients

1 bunch of spinach

bonito flakes

1 tsp of soy sauce

Directions

Boil spinach until it darkens. Rinse in cold water. Trim into 1-1/2 inch portions and squeeze excess water with your hands. Place in saucer, sprinkle with bonito flakes and soy sauce. Serve.

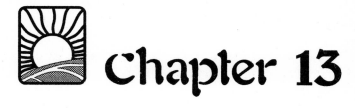

Chapter 13

Recipes

Day One Recipes

TEMPURA

(serves four)

8 large shrimp
4 small white fish filets
3 oz boneless chicken
2 bell peppers, quartered
1 Japanese eggplant, cut diagonally into thin strips
4 mushrooms

Tempura Batter
2 cups flour
1 cup chilled water
1 egg

Sauce
1 cup stock (see Chapter 12)
2T soy sauce
1t mirin sweet sake or pale dry sherry
1t sugar
5 oz daikon Japanese radish, finely grated
1/4 inch fresh ginger, peeled and finely shredded

Sprinkle chicken and peppers with salt and allow to stand.

Prepare batter by mixing egg and chilled water in a bowl. Sift flower over mixture and mix lightly (do not overmix or batter will become sticky).

Heat oil in a deep frying pan to about 340 degrees. Dry all ingredients, dip in batter and deep fry until golden brown. Drain on paper towel.

Serve with dipping sauce made by combining soup stock, sake, soy sauce and sugar. Serve ginger and daikon separately.

HIJIKI AND SESAME SEEDS
(serves one)

2/3 oz hijiki (seaweed)
1t sesame seeds
1 cup soup stock (see Chapter 12)
1t mirin sweet sake or pale dry sherry
2 sliced, peeled carrots
2 cakes deep fried tofu (abura-age), cut into strips
1/2t soy sauce
1/2t salad oil
1T sugar
dash of salt

Soak hijiki in water then strain. Heat oil in sauce pan. Stir-fry carrots and tofu. Add hijiki, soup stock, salt, sake and boil until stock is absorbed. Place in serving bowl, sprinkle with sesame seeds and serve.

WAKAME SOUP

(serves one)

3/4 oz wakame (dry curling seaweed)
3/4 cup soup stock (see Chapter 12)
4 slices of bamboo shoots
1t sake
1t salad oil
chopped green onion
salt and pepper

Rehydrate wakame and cut into 1-inch strips. Remove tough center vein if necessary. Bring stock to a boil, add bamboo shoots, sake, salad oil, salt and pepper. Add wakame, and green pepper. Bring to boil and serve immediately.

PORK AND POTATOES

(serves four)

6-1/2 oz lean pork, cut into thin, bite-sized pieces
8 new potatoes, peeled and cut into bite size pieces
2 onions, cut into thin wedges
soup stock (see Chapter 12)
4T soy sauce
3T sugar
2T sake

In a stew pot, heat oil and fry pork quickly. Add potatoes and onions. Add enough stock to barely cover meat. Add soy sauce, sugar and sake.

Cover and simmer until potatoes are done.

TOFU WITH DAIKON LEAVES
        (serves four)

Daikon greens, the tops from long Japanese radishes, make this dish high in calcium. Turnip leaves may be substituted.

2 cakes soft tofu, cut in 3/4-inch cubes
leaves from one daikon, cut into 2-inch lengths
3/4 oz shirasuboshi (dried white sardine)
2 eggs
1 cup soup stock
2T salad oil

Briefly boil shirasuboshi. Beat eggs and add sardines. Heat salad oil in a sauce pan and stir in leaves. Add soup stock, sake, sugar and soy sauce and bring to a boil. Add tofu and simmer over low flame.

When tofu is done, pour in egg mixture and immediately turn off flame.

Serve when eggs are soft boiled.

Day Two Recipes

PIZZA TOAST
(serves one)

1 oz frozen mixed vegetables
6 small frozen shrimp
1 slice bread
1/4t butter
1/2 oz mild white cheese

Thaw vegetables and shrimp. Arrange vegetables and shrimp on toast. Top with cheese and bake until cheese is melted.

BEEF, SHIRATAKI, AND TOFU
(serves one)

1-3/4 oz thinly-sliced lean beef, cut into bit-sized pieces
2-1/2 oz grilled tofu, cubed
1-1/2 oz shirataki (vermicelli-like threads) cut into short lengths
2 green onions, cut into small pieces lengthwise
snow peas
1/2 cup stock (see Chapter 12)
2 thin pieces of ginger root, finely chopped
2t mirin sweet sake or pale dry sherry
2t soy sauce

Bring stock to a boil. Add beef and ginger and simmer, skimming any foam.

Add grilled tofu, shirataki, sake, and soy sauce. Add snowpeas and boil briefly before serving.

DAIKON SALAD
(serves four)

6 oz daikon
5 oz carrots
4T lemon juice
2T soy sauce

Cut radish and carrots into thin strips.
Toss with lemon and soy sauce

BROCCOLI AND TOFU SOUP
(serves four)

1 bunch broccoli, cut into bite-size pieces
1/2 cake soft tofu, cut into 2-inch squares
3 cups stock (see Chapter 12)
pinch of salt
2t soy sauce
yuzu (citron) or lemon peel, shredded

Boil broccoli. In a sauce pan, combine stock, soy sauce and
salt. Add tofu and broccoli and simmer. Serve in Japanese-style
soup bowls topped with lemon

SARDINES IN UMEBOSHI SAUCE
(serves four)

8 fresh sardines, cleaned with heads removed
4 umeboshi (pickled plums)
6T soy sauce
1T sake
2T sugar

Mix 2/3 cup of water in sauce pan with soy sauce, sake, and
sugar and bring to a boil. Add sardines. When nearly done, add
umeboshi. Cook over a low flame, basting sauce over sardines
until the sauce has reduced by 2/3.

BRUSSEL SPROUTS AND CARROTS
(serves four)

10 oz small brussel sprouts
2 carrots, cut into bite-sized pieces
2T soy sauce
2T vinegar
3T salad oil
1/8-inch of fresh ginger, peeled and finely chopped.

Cook sprouts and carrots in salted water until done. Mix soy sauce, vinegar, oil and ginger and pour over hot vegetables, allowing flavors to blend a few minutes.

Day Three Recipes

FROZEN YOGURT AND FRUIT
(serves one)

1 cup plain yogurt
1/2 banana
1 kiwi fruit
4 strawberries

Cut fruit into small pieces. Blend into yogurt. Freeze, stirring occasionally.

BOILED BEANS WITH MUSHROOMS AND CARROTS
(serves four)

This is a high-nutrient, low calorie tasty dish. The soy beans must be soaked for about 10 hours before cooking.

3-1/2 oz soaked, dried soy beans
1/3 cake konnyaku (vegetable starch)
3 carrots
1 4-inch strip kombu (dried black kelp)
4 dried shiitake mushrooms or other mushrooms
2c soup stock(see Chapter 12)
1 T sugar
6T soy sauce
3T sake or dry sherry

Boil soaked beans until soft. Drain and set aside. Dice konnyaku, kombu, carrots and mushroons into small cubes about the size of beans.

Put vegetables and beans in boiling soup stock and cook over moderate flame. Add soy sauce, sugar and sake and serve.

BOILED SPINACH AND BEAN SPROUTS
(serves four)

1 bunch spinach, washed and cut into 1/2-inch lengths
6 oz bean sprouts
1T vinegar
1T soy sauce

Wash bean sprouts and boil 2-3 minutes. Rinse immediately in cold water to cool. Boil spinach 2 minutes, rinse in cold water and squeeze to remove excess water. Blend vegetables with vinegar and soy sauce and serve.

WAKAME AND TOFU MISO SOUP
(serves four)

4 cups basic stock (see Chapter 12)
5T miso (soybean paste)
1 package tofu
1/3 oz dried wakame (seaweed)

Add tofu and wakame to boiling stock

Dissolve miso in a bowl with some boiling stock. Stir into soup. Heat thoroughly and serve.

MACKEREL WITH TOMATO AND ONION DRESSING
(serves four)

1 lb mackerel, cleaned
3/4 onion, chopped
2 tomatoes, chopped
1 bell pepper, chopped
parsley
4T salad oil
1 cup stock (see Chapter 12)

1T white wine
1T vinegar
salt and pepper

Salt mackerel and set aside for 10 minutes. Heat salad oil in frying pan. Add fish and pour wine and vinegar over skin. Add soup and simmer until done

Transfer fish to serving plate and top with combined chopped vegetables.

TOFU AND VEGETABLE MIX
(serves four)

1/3 cake konnyaku (vegetable starch)
2 carrots, cut into matchstick-sized pieces
4T soup stock (see Chapter 12)
1T sake
1 cake tofu
1/2T salt
3T sugar
snowpeas
3 fresh shiitake mushrooms or other mushrooms, chopped
1t light soy sauce
1t sugar
1t white miso (shiro miso soybean paste)
1T mirin sweet sake or pale dry sherry
3T sesame seeds

Boil konnyaku and cut into 1-inch lengths the size of match sticks Combine carrots and mushrooms with soup, sake, soy sauce, and sugar and boil until soft. Boil snowpeas in salted water 1/2 minute. Cut diagonally.

Crush sesame seeds with mortar and pestle. Drain excess water from tofu by pressing against slanted board. Mix tofu, sesame seeds, salt, sugar, and sake. Drain vegetables and mix with tofu.

EGG AND LEEK SOUP

(serves four)

2 leeks
2 eggs, beaten
3 cups stock (see Chapter 12)
1t salt
1T soy sauce
1/2t sake

Cut off tough, outer green leaves, wash leeks thoroughly and cut into 1-inch strips. Boil three cups of stock, add salt, soy sauce, sake and leeks.

Drizzle eggs into soup, spiraling out to the edge of the pot. Serve immediately.

STEAMED CHICKEN

(serves one)

This dish can also be made with white fish topped with mushrooms and spinach

1/2 chicken breast, skinned
1/4 cup celery with leaves, sliced lengthwise into strips
1/4 onion, cut into small wedges
1 sliced clove of garlic
sake
salt and pepper
juice of 1/2 lemon

Place chicken on a large piece of aluminum foil. Shake on a dash of sake. Top with vegetables. Fold foil into a package and steam in a covered steamer for 15 minutes. Open, squeeze lemon on top and serve.

CREAMED BROCCOLI AND MUSHROOMS
(serves four)

16 fresh shiitake or other mushrooms, chopped
1 bunch broccoli, cut into bite size piecess
2 cups lowfat milk
1 egg yolk
1 cup stock (see Chapter 12)
2T flour
6T butter

Cook broccoli in boiling water. Saute mushrooms in 3T butter.

Add broccoli and toss. Make a white sauce by melting 3T butter in a sauce pan. Stir in flour then add milk to the paste.

Add the broccoli-mushroom mixture and simmer briefly. Stir in egg yolk and serve.

Day Four Recipes

YELLOWTAIL NABE
(serves four)

4 fillets yellowtail tuna cut into bite-sized pieces
1 lb daikon radish cut into half-moon shapes 1/2 inch thick
8 shiitake mushrooms
2 carrots, quartered and cut into 1-inch lengths
Four leaves of shungiku (green herb) Use only
    tender outer leaves
4 cups soup stock (see Chapter 12)
2T sake
3T soy sauce
scallions
salt and pepper

Salt fish and let stand for 5 minutes. Add to boiling water and
simmer until not quite done. Remove. Cut deep crosses in the
caps of the mushrooms. Set aside. Heat soup stock, add sake,
soy sauce and salt. Add fish, radish, carrots, and mushrooms.
When carrots are soft, add shungiku. Top with grated daikon
and slivered scallions and serve.

RED SNAPPER SOUP
(serves four)

6 oz red snapper or any other white fish,
    cut into bite-sized portions.
3 scallions, chopped
3 cup stock (see Chapter 12)
1/2t salt
1/2t sake
1t soy sauce
yuzu (citron) or lemon peel

Salt fish and let stand 10 minutes. Heat stock, add soy sauce,
sake and bring to boil. Add fish and boil until cooked. To serve,
put one portion of fish into a soup bowl, add stock and garnish
with scallions and lemon rind.

MABODOFU

(serves four)

This Chinese-style dish is very popular in Japan. It also may be made with beef, chicken or shrimp

2 cakes silk tofu, diced
3 oz ground pork
2 eggplant, sliced into discs
1 cup beef boullion
1/4 oz red miso (soybean paste)
dash soy sauce
chopped ginger to taste
1 clove garlic, peeled and chopped
7-spice chili powder to taste
2/3T sugar
cornstarch

Heat oil in a frying pan. Add ginger, garlic and tofu. Cook briefly. Add meat and eggplant and stir fry. Pour in soup, sake, soy sauce, sugar. Thicken with cornstarch if necessary. Add chili powder to taste.

SPINACH AND TUNA SALAD

(serves four)

1 bunch spinach
1 can tuna
1t soy sauce.

Coarsely chop spinach, boil one minute and drain thoroughly. Add tuna and mix. Dress with soy sauce.

CHICKEN AND CASHEW NUTS
(serves four)

2 skinned chicken breasts, cut into bite-sized pieces
3 oz cashews
1 small onion, chopped
5 oz bamboo shoots, chopped
2 bell peppers, seeded and chopped
1/4-inch slice ginger, peeled and chopped
3T soup stock (see Chapter 12)
2T salad oil
1t soy sauce
2t sake
1T cornstarch
salt and pepper

Mix chicken, soy sauce, sake, salt, pepper and cornstarch. Heat oil in frying pan and stir-fry onions and ginger. Add chicken mixture and cook. Pour in soup and bring to boil. Add vegetables and cook. Add cashews and serve.

STIR-FRIED CORN, PEAS, AND CHEESE
(serves four)

5-1/4 oz corn kernals
2T peas
3-1/2 oz cheese, cut into 1/2-inch squares
IT butter
1/2t sugar
salt and pepper

Boil corn and peas until done. Drain. Melt butter in heated sauce pan. Add corn and peas and toss. Add remaining ingredients and cook until cheese is melted.

Day Five Recipes

SQUID, SHRIMP AND BROCCOLI
(serves four)

1 head broccoli, cut into bite-sized pieces
3 oz squid, cut into pieces
8 shrimp, shelled
4 fresh shiitake mushrooms, cut in half
1/2-inch ginger, peeled and chopped
3T salad oil
1 cup soup stock (see Chapter 12)
1t sugar
salt and pepper

Boil broccoli and drain. Heat oil in a sauce or frying pan. Stir-fry fish, mushrooms and broccoli. Add soup, sake, salt and sugar and boil for 2 minutes. Serve.

CARROT SALAD
(serves four)

Four large carrots, cut into thin strips
1/2 cup raisins
1/2 onion, sliced into thin rings
1T soy sauce
1T vinegar
Lettuce.

Soak raisins in hot water to plump. Combine all ingredients. Line individual bowls with lettuce leaf and top with carrot mixture.

SUKIYAKI

(serves four)

1-1/2 lb thinly-sliced beef
1 package (10-1/2 oz) grilled tofu
1/4 lb shungiku (green herb)
5 leaves of Chinese cabbage, cut into bite-sized pieces
1 onion, cut into small wedges
2 scallions, cut diagonally into 1 1/2-inch pieces
6 shiitake mushrooms
shirataki (shredded vermicelli-like threads)

Broth
1/2 cup stock (see Chapter 12)
3T sugar
1T sweet sake or pale dry sherry
1/2c soy sauce

Heat metal casserole, preferably one you can take to the table as a serving bowl, with oil. Add beef and fry quickly. Add onions and cook. Pour in broth and heat. Add tofu and mushrooms. Add cabbage and shungiku.
Serve from casserole.

VINEGARED DAIKON AND CARROTS

(serves four)

1 lb daikon, cut in thin strips
4 carrots, cut in thin strips
juice from 1/2 lemon
5T vinegar
2t sugar

Sprinkle carrots and daikon with salt and let stand. Squeeze out excess water. Add vinegar, sugar, and lemon juice. Cover with a heavy weight and let stand 30 minutes to blend flavors.

Day Six Recipes

EGG-CHEESE OMELETTE
(serves four)

1/2 chicken breast, cut into pieces
4 raw shiitake mushrooms
1 small onion, coarsely chopped
1 bell pepper, seeded and coarsely chopped
8 eggs
3 oz mozzerella cheese, shredded
parsley
tabasco
ketchup
2T salad oil

Each omelette serving is made individually. For each serving: put 1/2t oil in frying pan. Beat two eggs and add to pan. Top with 1/4 of cheese, chicken, mushrooms, onions, and pepper. Cover and cook until chicken is done. Add parsley, tabasco or ketchup to taste.

PORK AND SWEET POTATOES
(Serves four)

6-1/2 oz lean pork, cut into bite-sized pieces
1 small sweet potato, cut into bite-sized pieces
1/3 oz wakame (seaweed)
2T salad oil
1-1/2 c stock (see Chapter 12)
2T sake
2T sugar
2T soy sauce
1T mirin sweet sake or pale dry sherry

Rehydrate wakame and cut into bite-sized pieces. Stir-fry pork in oil. Add sweet potatoes and coat with oil. Add sugar, soy sauce and stock. On medium heat, cover and simmer until potatoes are soft. Add sake and wakame. Bring to boil and serve.

DAIKON, CARROTS, AND CUCUMBER SALAD
(Serves four)

6 oz daikon, cut into thin strips
2 carrots, cut into thin strips
1 cucumber, cut into strips
juice from 1/2 lemon
1T soy sauce
1T white sesame seeds

Toss vegetables in a bowl. Top with sesame seeds and dress with lemon and soy sauce.

SALMON SAUTE
(Serves four)

4 salmon steaks
2T flour
1 egg, beaten
1T butter
1T oil
8 raw shiitake or other mushrooms, cut in half
2 bell peppers, cut into bite-sized pieces
1 lemon

Heat butter and oil in frying pan. Sprinkle salmon with salt and pepper. Dredge in flour and dip in beaten egg. Fry salmon until done. Remove salmon and saute mushrooms and peppers in the frying pan. Serve steaks on individual plates with vegetables and lemon wedge.

SPINACH AND BEAN SPROUTS SAUTEED
(serves four)

1 bunch spinach, chopped into 2-inch pieces
3/4 lb bean sprouts
1T salad oil
salt and pepper

Boil spinach 2 minutes. Plunge into cold water, drain and squeeze out excess water. Wash bean sprouts and shake off excess water. Heat oil in a frying pan and stir fry bean sprouts and spinach. Add salt and pepper.

Day Seven Recipes

GAMMODOKI, SHIITAKE AND VEGETABLES
(serves four)

12 small gammodoki (cod cakes)
8 shiitake or other mushrooms
12 string beans
2-1/2 cups stock (see Chapter 12)
4T sugar
3T soy sauce
2T mirin sake or pale dry sherry

In a strainer, wash gammodoki in hot water and drain. In sauce pan, bring stock to boil. Add mushrooms and gammodoki. Add sugar, sake, soy sauce and heat to blend flavors. Add string beans and simmer until done.

CHICKEN AND CHINESE CABBAGE
(serves four)

Two chicken breasts, cut into pieces
Small head Chinese cabbage
5 shiitake or other dry mushrooms
5 oz bamboo shoots
3T sake
1T sugar
3T soy sauce
1 thin slice ginger, chopped
1T cornstarch
1T salad oil

Rehydrate mushrooms by soaking them in hot water for 15 minutes. Cut into quarters. Cut bamboo shoots and cabbage into bite-sized pieces. Heat oil in sauce pan and stir-fry chicken. Add vegetables, sake, soy sauce, sugar and ginger. Cook until done. Thicken with cornstarch if necessary.

OKARA

(serves four)

1 lb okara (byproduct of making tofu)
1/2 cup green onions, cut into strips
3 oz clams, shrimp or other shellfish, shelled
2 slices kamaboko (fish cake) cut into strips
1/2 carrot cut into strips
2 shiitake mushrooms

Heat oil in frying pan. Fry clams. Add vegetables and stir. Add okara. Add sake, sugar, soy sauce and cook, stirring, for 2 to 3 minutes more until done.

FISH CASSEROLE

(serves four)

7 oz red snapper, cut into pieces
4 oz squid, cut into pieces
8 shrimp, shelled
4 clams
12 oysters
1 carrot, thinly sliced
2 scallions
5 leaves of Chinese cabbage, cut into serving pieces
1 cake soft tofu
4 shiitake mushrooms
1/4 lb shungiku (green herb)
13 oz udon noodles
soup stock (see Chapter 12)

In a casserole, preferably one that can be used as a serving bowl, boil soup stock, adding soy sauce, sake, and thick cabbage stems. Add fish, tofu and other vegetables. When fish is done, add oysters and shrimp.

In Japan, diners pick out the food with chopsticks from the boiling stew. At the end of the meal, the udon noodles are added to the boiling stock with whatever vegetables are left and then eaten from the pot.

Other Recipes from the Japanese Table

Casseroles

ODEN

(serves four)

This nutritious, popular casserole often is served in the cool autumn months and can be a meal in itself. It uses a variety of ingredients made from tofu. Oden often includes a hard boiled egg with the shell removed. Although all ingredients listed here may not be used each time, it is common to include 6 or 10. Most ingredients can be purchased prepackaged in Japanese food stores.

2 cakes deep-fried tofu (atsu-age)
1 cake konnyaku (vegetable paste)
16 string beans
8 inches of daikon radish, shredded
12 ginko nuts
4 strips kombu (kelp)
4 cabbage leaves
1 chikuwa (grilled fish paste rolls)
4 satsuma-age balls (fried fish balls)
4 shrimp wrapped with abura-age
4 octopus tentacles

CABBAGE ROLLS
4 cabbage leaves
3-1/2 oz ground chicken
1 small onion, chopped
1 oz bamboo shoots, chopped

BROTH
7 cups stock (see chapter 12)
1/3 c light soy sauce
2T sugar
3T mirin (sweet sake, or pale dry sherry)

Tie the kombu strips in knots and place in the bottom of the casserole. Add stock and bring to a boil. Immediately reduce to a low flame and add sugar, soy sauce, sake. Stir in vegetables and konnyaku. Bring to a boil again and then simmer for 10 minutes. Add the tofu products. Finally, add fish and meat. Cover and simmer for about an hour. Diners help themselves from the casserole.

To make the cabbage rolls: mix the chicken, onions and bamboo shoots. Drop cabbage leaves in boiling water to soften, then wrap the chicken mixture in individual leaves. Tie with kampyo (edible gourd shavings) or tie with a string. Add rolls to simmering stock with other meat ingredients.

CHICKEN MIZUTAKI

(serves four)

3/4 pound of chicken cut into bite-sized pieces
5 leaves of Chinese cabbage, cut into 2-inch lengths
1 cake of tofu cut into one-inch cubes
8 snow peas
bamboo shoots
1 lb. daikon radish
1 square of kombu (kelp)

Wipe kombu with a clean towel and place in the bottom of a casserole. Top with chicken. Add enough water to cover the chicken and bring to a boil. When it begins to boil, remove kelp and skim any foam from top of water. Lower flame and simmer for about 40 minutes, or until chicken is tender. Add tofu and vegetablese and simmer until tender. Serve from casserole.

BOILED TOFU AND KOMBU (KELP)
(serves four)

3 cakes of tofu
6-inch square of kombu (kelp)
1/3 c stock (see chapter 12)
1/3 c mirin (sweet sake or pale dry sherry)
2/3 c of soy sauce
a small chunk of ginger, grated
1/3 onion

Cut tofu into 2-inch cubes. Snip kombu at the sides in 2 or 3 places. Cut onion into thin strips. Mix the stock, mirin, soy sauce and ginger and bring to a boil in a sauce pan. In a ceramic casserole, place kombu on the bottom, add a small amount of water and tofu. When mixture boils, add stock mixture from sauce pan. Simmer.

CLAMS AND VEGETABLES WITH MUSTARD/VINEGAR AND MISO DRESSING
(serves four)

1/2 pound clams (any small clam may be used or substitute small pieces of chicken)
4 green onions
bamboo shoots
1/3 oz wakame (curly dried seaweed)
2-1/2 ounces white miso
2t mustard
3T rice vinegar
1T sugar

If clams are fresh, cook and loosen from shell or simmer chicken until tender. Drop onions in boiling water until they turn bright green and are lightly cooked. Remove, rinse in cold water and cut into 1-inch-long strips. Rehydrate wakame and cut into 1-inch strips. Boil briefly. Using only the top soft part of the bamboo shoot, cut into thin pieces and boil briefly. In a small bowl, combine mustard, vinegar and miso topping. Arrange vegetables and clams on a platter. Top with mustard mixture.

CHICKEN AND GRATED DAIKON

(serves four)

1 pound daikon radish
1 cucumber
1 stalk celery
3 radishes
1/2 pound skinned chicken breast
one lemon
1T soy sauce

Salt chicken and season with sake. Steam until tender. Cool and tear into bite-sized pieces. Grate daikon and drain out excess water. Cut celery and cucumber into thin slices. Combine radish, celery and cucumber with chicken in a bowl.

Make the dressing by combining soy sauce and lemon juice. Serve dressing in individual bowls. Guests take chicken from the serving bowl and add their own dressing.

Fish Dishes

STEAMED SEA BREAM AND KOMBU

(serves one)

4 oz sea bream or other firm, white fish
1 sheet kombu (seaweed)
3 long stems of mitsuba, with leaves
Yuzu (citron) or lemon peel

Wipe kombu with towel and place in bottom of bowl. Season fish with salt and sake and steam for about 15 minutes. During last 5 minutes of steaming, add mitsuba and yuzu peel.

SALMON OCHAZUKE
(Serves four)

Ochazuke is a rice/soup dish that is quick and nutritious. It is especially satisfying in the cold winter months as a light meal when a plain bowl of rice may not quite hit the spot. Salmon, pollock roe or umeboshi are commonly used.

1 oz baked, salted salmon
1 cup cooked rice
1 cup soup (see chapter 12)
dash of salt
1T sake
2 sheets of nori cut into thin strips
sesame seeds if desired

Remove skin and bones from salmon, tear into small chunks. Add salt and sake to stock and bring to a boil. Put rice in a bowl and top with cut nori. Sprinkle with sesame seeds if desired and top with salmon. Top with a 1/4-inch cube of wasabi (Japanese horseradish) and pour hot soup into the bowl. Cover with a lid and serve.

YELLOWTAIL TERIYAKI
(serves four)

4 pieces of yellowtail tuna
4T soy sauce
4T mirin (sweet sake or dry pale sherry)
2-3T sugar

In a small sauce pan, bring soy, mirin and sugar to a boil. Turn off heat. Bake the fish. When it begins to change color, baste with sauce and turn. Repeat, turning fish twice.

Meat Dishes

ROLLED BEEF
(Serves four)

3/4 pound thinly-cut beef
1/2 carrot
20 string beans
2T soy sauce
2T mirin (sweet sake or pale, dry sherry)
2T salad oil

String beans and cut them and carrots into long strips. Boil briefly. Spread meat and season with salt and pepper. Wrap carrots and string beans in beef. Heat oil in frying pan and stir fry, adding mirin and soy sauce to flavor. When done, cut into one-inch pieces and serve.

BOILED CHICKEN MIXED WITH VEGETABLES
(serves four)

7 ounces skinless chicken breast
7 ounces bamboo shoots
3 carrots
3 oz renkon (lotus root)
1 cake konnyaku (vegetable paste)
4 dried shiitake mushrooms
10 snow peas
2 cups soup stock (see chapter 12)
1T salad oil
2T sugar
3T soy sauce
1T mirin (sweet sake or dry, pale sherry)

Cut chicken into bite sized pieces. Peel carrots and lotus root and cut into bite-sized bits. Cut bamboo shoots into bite-sized pieces. Cut konnyaku into bite-sized pieces and boil briefly. Rehydrate mushrooms and cut into pieces. String snowpeas and boil quickly in salted water until bright green. In frying pan, heat salad oil and stir-fry chicken. Remove chicken to a dish and add soy sauce, mirin and sugar. Add carrots, bamboo shoots, lotus root, konnyaku and mushrooms to the frying pan and stir fry. Add soup stock, sugar, soy sauce and mirin. Simmer for 20 minutes. Add chicken and stir. Cook until water evaporates. Add snow peas and serve.

PORK AND TOFU

(serves four)

7 ounces of thinly-sliced pork
2 cakes tofu
1 green onion
3-1/2 ounces of shirataki (noodles)
1 bunch spinach
1 cup soup stock (see chapter 12)
2T sugar
3T soy sauce
1T sake
1T salad oil
1 small slice chopped ginger

Cut pork into bite-sized bits. Season with soy sauce and ginger. Cut tofu into 10 pieces. Cut noodles into short pieces, boil briefly and drain. Cut spinach into 1-inch strips and cook briefly. Drain. In frying pan, heat oil and stir fry pork. When it changes color, add sugar, soy sauce and sake. Add other ingredients except spinach. Add soup stock until all ingredients are covered. Simmer until tofu absorbs the flavor. Add spinach and serve.

■

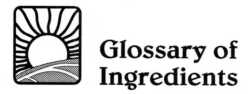

Glossary of Ingredients

In a few cases, items found in a Western kitchen may be substituted but many Japanese recipes call for special ingredients found in a well-stocked Japanese market or occasionally in American grocery stores.

Abura-Age — deep fried tofu puffs made from soybean milk.

Chikuwa — ground white fish meat made into a paste and either steamed or grilled.

Daikon — A Japanese white radish. Much bigger and milder than common red radishes. The tops may be eaten as a green vegetable.

Daizu — Dried soybeans.

Dashi no moto — Instant mix for basic soup stock available packaged in many forms.

Gammodoki — Dumpling-like cakes made of cod fish and vegetables. Available packaged at Japanese markets.

Hakusai — Chinese cabbage or substitute Napa cabbage

Hijiki — A form of seaweed. Available packaged.

Kamaboko — steamed fish paste formed into cakes.

Kampyo — Strips of dried, edible gourd used for tying food. Before using, soak in salt water, rinse and boil until soft.

Katsuobushi — Dried bonito. Available packaged in Japanese markets.

Kombu — Dried kelp. Sold packaged in Japanese markets.

Konnyaku — Hard, translucent loaf made from vegetable starch.

Koya-dofu — freeze-dried tofu. Soak in lukewarm water until soft before cooking.

Mirin — Sweet sake used for cooking. Pale dry sherry may be substituted, or regular sake sweetened.

Miso — Soybean paste used as flavoring for soup or as a dressing for vegetables. Available packaged in Japanese groceries. Miso soup mix, including miso and some vegetables, is available packaged.

Okara — A by-product of the process of making tofu. Available fresh in Japanese markets.

Saba — Japanese mackerel. Any type of mackerel or firm white fish like snapper may be substituted.

Satsuma-age balls — balls of kamaboko which have been deep fried

Shiitake — Japanese mushrooms available dried. Reconstitute by soaking in water for 30 minutes.

Shirasuboshi — Dried small sardines. Available in Japanese groceries.

Shirataki — Shredded vermicelli-like threads available in Japanese markets. Made from a vegetable starch, not wheat.

Shungiku — A green herb translated as chrysanthemum leaves. It is not the leaf of the commonly-grown flower.

Tofu — Custard-like cake made of soybean curd. Sold fresh in Japanese markets. Regular tofu is strained with cheescloth. Finer, softer version is strained through silk.

Umeboshi — Small pickled plums available in Japanese markets.

Wakame — Curly, dried seaweed. Available dried in packages.

Yakidofu — Grilled tofu. Available packaged.

Yuzu — Citrus fruit like citron. Available packaged in Japanese groceries. Lemon peel may be substituted.

■

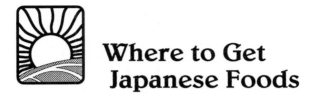

Where to Get Japanese Foods

If your local supermarket doesn't stock some of the foods listed is this book, you should be able to find them at an oriental market. Health or natural food stores and gourmet shops also carry many items of Japanese food.

The following list includes some other sources. Some of these firms sell food by mail. The importers and manufacturers on the list generally do not sell food directly, but they can give you the names of retailers in your area who carry their products.

Arkansas
Mountain Ark Trading Co.   (800) 643-8909
120 S.East Street   Mailorder
Fayetteville, AR 72701

California
House of Rice   (916) 893-1794
338 Broadway   Retail
Chico, CA 95928

Japan Food Corporation   (415) 873-8400
445 Kaufman Court   Importer
San Francisco, CA 94080

Japantown Foods   (408) 255-7980
5289-F Prospect Rd.   Retail
San Jose, CA 95129

Nishimoto Trading Co., Ltd.
1111 Mateo St.   (213) 689-9330
Los Angeles, CA 90021   Importer

Nishimoto Trading Co.,Ltd.   (415) 871-2490
410 East Grand Ave.   Importer
South San Francisco, CA 94080

Ohsawa America   (800) 647-2929
P.O. Box 12717, Northgate Station Importer
San Rafael, CA 94913

San-J International   (415) 821-4040
384 Liberty   Manufacturer
San Francisco, CA 94114

Westbrae Natural Foods   (213) 722-1692
4240 Hollis Street   Manufacturer
Emeryville, CA 94608

Colorado
East-West Gifts   (303) 493-0808
203 West Myrtle   Mailorder
Fort Collins, CO 80521

Florida
Tree of Life, Inc.   (904) 824-8181
P.O. Box 410   Manufacturer
St. Augustine, FL 32084

Illinois
Toguri Mercantile Co.   (312) 929-3500
851 W. Belmont Ave.   Retail
Chicago, IL 60657

Maryland
Sakura Oriental Books & Food   (301) 468-0605
15809 South Frederick Rd.   Retail
Rockville, MD 20855

Michigan
Eden Foods   (517) 456-7424
701 Tecumseh Rd.   Importer, ask for customer
Clinton, MI 49236   service

New Jersey
Edward & Sons   (201) 964-8176
P.O. Box 3150   Importer
Union, NJ 07083

Nishimoto Trading Co. Ltd.   (212) 349-0056
21-23 Empire Blvd.   Importer
South Hackensack, NJ 07606

Nebraska
Aki Oriental Foods & Gifts   (402) 339-2671
4425 So. 84th Street   Retail
Omaha, NE 68127

New York
The Kimms   (914) 331-3999
316 Wall Street   Retail
Kingston, NY 12401

Oregon
Anzen Pacific Corp.   (503) 283-1284
P.O. Box 11407   Retail, Mailorder
Portland, OR 97211

Import Plaza   (503) 227-4050
#1 N.W. Couch St.   Retail, 21 stores throughout
Portland, OR 97209   Oregon

Washington
Granum   (206) 525-0051
2901 NE Blakely St.   Retail, mailorder
Seattle, WA 98105

Uwajimaya   (206) 624-6248
6th So. & So. King   Retail 3 stores, mailorder
Seattle, WA 98104

■

Charts

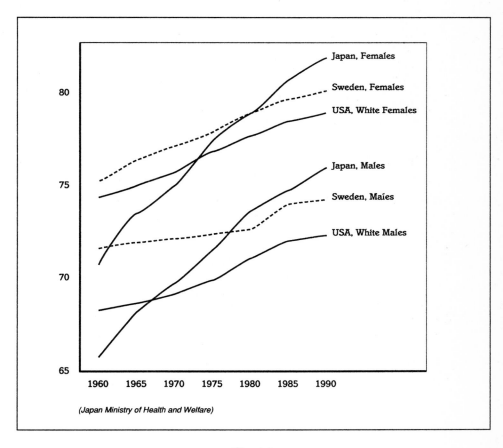

Chart 1
Increase in average life-span since 1960 in Japan, Sweden and the U.S.

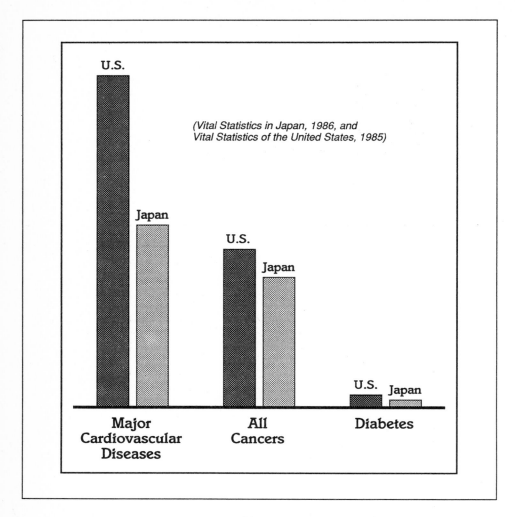

Chart 2

Comparison of death rates for heart disease, cancer and
diabetes in the U.S. and Japan

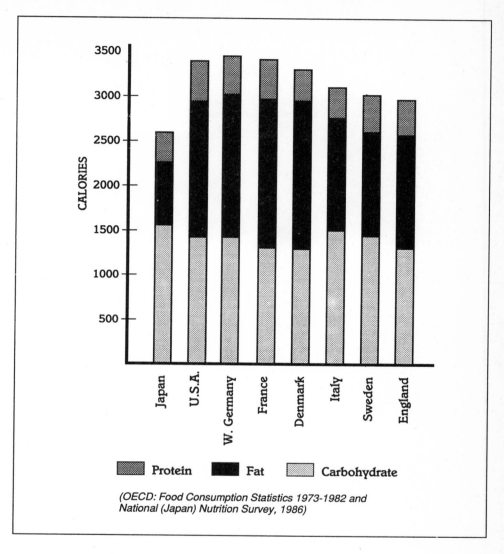

Chart 3

Caloric intake, total and of protein, fats, and
carbohydrates in selected countries

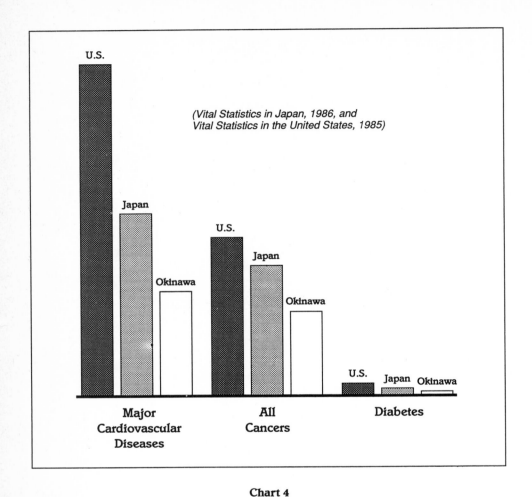

Chart 4
Okinawa has an exceptionally healthy population as illustrated by
these figures which compare the death rates for three of the
major causes of death in the United States, Japan, and Okinawa.

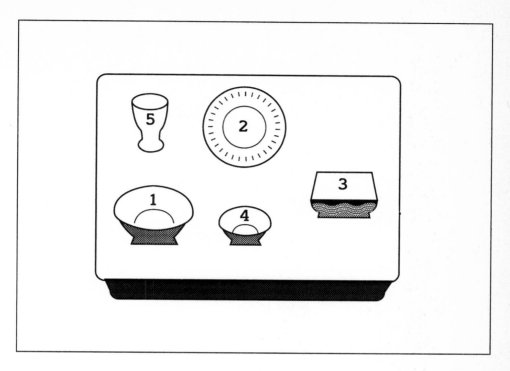

Chart 5

The Japanese Meal
1. rice
2. the main entry
3. the side dishes
4. soup
5. green tea.

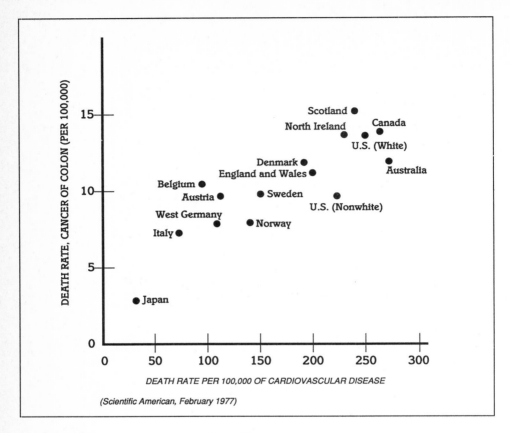

Chart 6

The apparent correlation between cancer of the colon rates
and cardiovascular disease suggests common, probably
dietary, causes. Both are far higher for Western
countries than for Japan.

Chart 7
Vitamin content of soybeans and soybean productsd per 100 grams.

	A I.U.	B$_1$ mg	B$_2$ mg	Niacin mg	C mg
edame	60	0.32	0.16	1.3	3.0
dried	0	0.22	0.09	2.1	0
natto	0	0.07	0.56	1.1	0
miso	0	0.12	0.18	2.3	0
tofu	0	0.1	0.04	0.2	0
okara	0	0.11	0.04	0.3	0

Chart 8

Mineral content of soybeans and soybean productsd per 100 grams.

	Calcium mg	magnesium mg	selenium mg	iron mg
edame	70	285	30	1.7
dried	230	265	28	2.1
natto	90	240	35	3.3
miso	40	90	0	1.7
tofu	130	110	0	1.4
okara	100	90	0	1.2

Chart 9

Vitamin content of seaweed per 100 grams.

	A I.U.	B_1 mg	B_2 mg	Niacin mg	C mg
wakame	780	0.11	0.14	10.0	15
konbu	430	0.21	0.32	1.8	11
hijiki	310	0.0	10.14	1.8	0
nori	14,000	1.15	3.40	9.8	20

Chart 10
Mineral content of seaweed per 100 grams.

	Calcium mg	magnesium mg	selenium mg	iron mg
wakame	1,300	3,050	5.9	13
konbu	1,050	1,670	3.5	15
hijiki	1,400	2,360	4,6	55
nori	390	2,040	1.3	12

Chart 11

Vitamin content of lean pork and beef per 100 grams.
Nutritionally, pork is superior to beef.

	A I.U.	B_1 mg	B_2 mg	Niacin mg	C mg
pork	0	1.34	0.32	6.4	2
pork liver	43,000	0.34	3.60	14.0	20
beef	17	0.07	0.19	5.8	1
beef liver	40,000	0.22	3.00	13.5	30

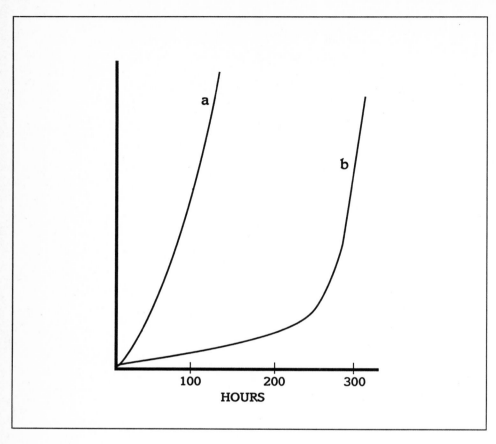

Chart 12
Development of rancidity in cooking oil when exposed to air.
(a) Untreated (b) Vitamin E added. Notice that even if the oil is treated
with vitamin E, it rapidly becomes rancid after about 10 days.

Index

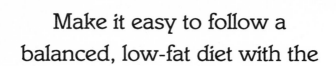

Make it easy to follow a
balanced, low-fat diet with the

East Meets West
Nutrition Planner
Computer Program.

It's hard to make sure that you and your family are getting the right balance of vitamins, minerals, proteins, carbohydrates, and fats for good health and long life. It's particularly hard to know how your diet is doing over the long term.

The East Meets West Nutrition Planner is designed to make getting good nutrition over the long term easy.

The Nutrition Planner is a computer program that calculates and stores not only the calories, but all the key nutrients for good health.

With it, you can determine the nutritional value of one meal or save and keep track of the nutritional value of your meals over a period of weeks, months, or years. You can readily identify what specific vitamins and minerals your diet lacks, and whether fat or salt may be in excess. You can follow your progress to a healthier diet and make corrections along the way.

The Nutrition Planner contains a large data base of both Japanese and Western foods. You just record what

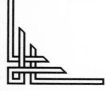

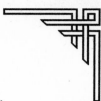
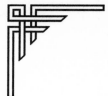

you've eaten. The computer does all the calculations and record keeping for you.

You can add new food items to the data base. The Nutrition Planner will learn and save the nutritional values for new recipes you give it.

Save the personal meal history of an unlimited number of individuals. Your whole family can benefit.

As of June 1989, the East Meets West Nutrition Planner is available only for IBM PC and compatible computers with 512K RAM and at least one floppy drive. The program can be copied to hard disk for greater ease of use.

Ask your local bookseller for the East Meets West Nutrition Planner or order directly from Ishi Press by sending $49.95 plus $3 shipping and handling to

Ishi Press International
1400 North Shoreline Boulevard, Bldg. A-7
Mountain View, CA 94043

Be sure to specify 5-1/4" or 3-1/2" diskette.

Start planning a
healthier diet today!

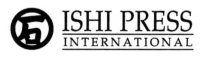

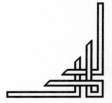
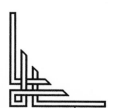